Journey into
the Heart of Bipolarity

An Artistic Point of View

Journey into the Heart of Bipolarity

An Artistic Point of View

Philippe Nuss
Marie Sellier
Jean-Paul Bath

John Libbey Eurotext Publishing

ISBN : 2-7420-0578-1

Éditions John Libbey Eurotext
127, avenue de la République
92120 Montrouge, France
Tel: 01 46 73 06 60
e-mail: contact@jle.com
http://www.jle.com

Editor: Maud Thévenin

© Éditions John Libbey Eurotext, 2005

It is prohibited to reproduce this work or any part of it without authorisation of the publisher or of the Centre Français d'Exploitation du Droit de Copie (CFC),
20, rue des Grands-Augustins, 75006 Paris.

Authors

Philippe Nuss

Dr Philippe Nuss, instigator and co-ordinator of this book project, is a psychiatrist in charge of the unit for first episode of psychosis and mood disorder at Saint-Antoine University Hospital Centre in Paris. He teaches at the Pierre et Marie Curie School of Medicine. He holds a special interest in educational principles and methods, whether addressed to students and care-givers or related to the psychoeducation of the patients and their families. His basic-research activity in structural and functional biology at the French Institute of Health and Medical Research, the INSERM (U538) involves studying the anomalies of membrane traffic in schizophrenia. He is an active member of a number of scholarly societies: International Society for Bipolar Disorders, Schizophrenia International Research Society, International Early Psychosis Association and the *Société Française de psychiatrie biologique*. He participates in many work groups on schizophrenia and bipolar disorder. Dr Nuss is also an expert for the French Health Regulation Authority.

Marie Sellier

A graduate of the Institut d'Études Politiques of Paris, Marie Sellier was a journalist for nearly fifteen years before moving into publishing. Having a passion for art, she started her first collection "*L'enfance de l'art*" in 1991 at Réunion des musées nationaux publisher. The collection today comprises eighteen books, most of which she has authored, and has been followed by another collection for the same publisher, "*Des mains pour créer*", at Éditions Paris-musées and "*Entrée libre*" at Éditions Nathan. She has written more than forty books favouring a sensitive approach of art and of the artists. Since 2000, she has combined art and fiction in children's books, including *L'Afrique, petit Chaka*, which sold more than 100,000 copies and won several awards. She imagined several books with the close involvement of contemporary painters: Marion Lesage, Luc Gauthier and Diagne Chanel. Her books have been translated into English, German, Spanish, Portuguese, Italian and Korean. Marie Sellier lives and works in Nogent-sur-Marne, in the greater Paris area.

Jean-Paul Bath

A defrocked engineer, Jean-Paul Bath was to prefer Pompidou Centre display areas to oil platforms. After nearly twenty years at the service of communication and the arts, with an MBA in his pocket he started up the firm Art Actuel, pooling the famous contemporary-art magazine of the same name and a consulting firm in communication through art, which organises exhibitions for its advertisers.

Contents

Foreword V

Introduction: A Clinical Gaze on the Sensitive 1

Bipolar Disorder in 1854: A Description 18

Bipolar Disorder: A Single Illness with Many Faces 32

The Bipolar's Palette 42

Mixed States 54

Key Data on Bipolarity 66

Bipolarity and Society? 74

References 83

Index of Artists 84

Psychiatry Index 86

Photo Credits 89

Acknowledgments 91

Graphic design: Jean-Marie Hoffschir

Translation: Marina Urquidi

Cover: Chia, Sandro: The Idleness of Sisyphus (1981). New York, Museum of Modern Art (MoMA). © Adagp, Paris 2005 – © 2005, Photo Scala, Florence. Oil on canvas, in two parts, 309.88 x 386.71 cm. Acquired through the Carter Burden, Barbara Jakobson, and Saidie A. May Funds and purchase.

Foreword

Our moods largely determine our subjective experience – how we feel about ourselves and the world in general. Bipolar mood disorder implies extremes – both up and down. Such extremes impose, on the many millions of people who suffer with bipolarity, subjective experiences that are out of the ordinary and objective problems that may be incapacitating. As a psychiatrist, I struggle to understand the objective problems and to describe the consistent clinical features of bipolar patients. By doing so, I believe we make possible a kind of consistency, in both diagnosis and treatment, which is essential for reliable knowledge, for a scientific psychiatry. I make no apology for that. However, I can also acknowledge the unique, the personal, the subjective in bipolar experience. Good clinical practice always connects with our patients' experiences. Moreover, we know that sometimes the experiences of people living with bipolar disorder are turned into art, which is puzzling and interesting, because most of us know relatively little about art, except what we like, of course. Philippe Nuss invites us to go further – to try and get at the subjective experience of bipolarity in a novel and intriguing way, through the work of visual artists he admires. He argues that the kind of emotional knowledge we get from art offers a novel dimension to our understanding of mood disorder - that a subjective understanding of the unique experiences of patients may be derived from those ingredients that constitute the universal appeal of great art. His appeal is to our imagination – how can we not want to read on!

GUY GOODWIN
Oxford, September 2005

A Clinical Gaze on the Sensitive

Why this book?

The book you are holding is out of the ordinary. Art book or a clinical manual for psychiatry, it is both of these and neither at the same time. It has chosen an uncommon angle: to describe different subjectivities – those inherent to works of art and the patients', both of these related to the readers' subjectivity. The expected effect is to bring about an understanding of the mental world of bipolar patients through a subtle play of correspondences in the interweaving of these three types of subjectivity.

This work was born from a clinical fact: patients' subjective perception is the reality on which they base the development of the main lines of their life plan. In psychiatric care, a patient's subjectivity is thus the starting point of his therapeutic process, of his acknowledgment that he is suffering from some form of disorder and of his consent to treatment. Subjectivity, an individual perception of the world, is a complex experience that is different for every patient and also changes as time goes by. It is understandable that doctors, when having to describe bipolar patients and to organise their disorder, have attempted to minimise in their symptomatology the subjectivity factor – because of its changing and unpredictable nature – to the benefit of reproducible, invariable and, most of all, easily observable manifestations. Description of the disorders has therefore progressively replaced the description of the patients. This approach is indispensable and legitimate, and, in fact, the very foundation of medical nosography. Nonetheless, not only does it deprive clinicians of the comprehension of the subjective forces that will move the patient and guide him through the treatment, it also removes them from another clinic, in our view equally important: the one that deals with what the patient experiences.

There is no denying that the psychopathological processes of mania or depression deeply change what patients experience. This latter, despite the constraint inherent to the disorder, remains nonetheless subjective. The constraint imposed by the disorder is twofold. On the one hand, it reduces the number of subjective states that patients can feel when they are well and on the other, it restricts those that they can experience potentially. Thus, for instance, patients who are depressed no longer have access, as they did previously, to pleasant subjective states and the subjective states that remain possible to them are submitted to the influence of the pessimism intrinsic to depression. This raises the question of how to get the most exact and relevant account of the changes that occur. The verbal description of subjective states is often limited because language, which is a coded system, is ill-suited to a concise description of subjective states. The idea was therefore to find mediators liable to account for both the patient's infinite possibilities of expression and the constraints imposed by the disorder. Using works of art as mediators for clinical understanding then appeared to us as being likely to achieve this. A work of art is, in fact, both subjective and constrained. It is subjective as much by the interpretation it provokes as by the emotion it inspires. It is constrained by the finished materiality of its plastic representation in fixed spatial and temporal dimensions, by the materials that constitute it and by the more-or-less explicit intention of the artist. Although it leaves the door open to a multiplicity of experiences, the work of art in fact constrains those who view it into a sensory and conceptual organisation. It is in this duality that we felt the work of art was apt to help understand the subjectivity of patients submitted to the constraints of their pathology. Finally, subjectivity also prevailed in our choices – our choices of bipolar clinical dimensions, as well as our choices of the art works that we selected. Other clinicians, other authors might have made different choices. Thus, far from being closed and from aiming at exhaustiveness, this book is designed to offer openings. The horizons of these openings will be seen in their own way by different clinicians, depending on their sensitivity and their practice.

Not exclusively reserved to clinicians, this book is also intended for everyone. Indeed, it seems important that the broadest public should be alerted to the fact that the subjective movements of the mental life of bipolar patients have their specificity, which is just as worthy of interest as it generates suffering. We also hope that a sensitive reading of this book will help bipolar patients and the people in their familiar circles to acquire a better understanding of the nature of their disorder and, on that basis, to contribute more favourably to the care that is offered.

A lunatic artist? A brilliant lunatic? Neither one!
Works of art devoted to the illustration of mental pathologies usually consider the subject from two perspectives. The first proposes to illustrate with the help of artistic iconography some of the clinical features of the disorder, such as for instance the sadness, the excitement, the anguish, the guilt, the delusion or the changes in body expressions caused by mental disorder. It proposes to exemplify, by virtue of a supposed analogy between the clinical aspect and the subject of the work, the observed aspects of the mental category involved, which in our case is bipolar disorder. The other approach of this type of

work is less descriptive. It presupposes a part of madness in all artists and a part of creative genius in all mental patients. In fact, this is the assumption that lays the foundations of Art Brut. Many people think, somewhat ingenuously, that because Van Gogh, Goya and Munch suffered from mental disorder, they illustrated, almost magnified in their work some of the psychopathological characteristics of the disorder from which they suffered.

We feel that these perspectives are debatable for two reasons.

The first reason disputes the existence of a potential and almost mandatory link between madness and creativeness. Indeed, a common denominator to all mental pathologies (this would also apply to somatic pathologies) lies precisely in their unchangeable character, their fixed nature, which makes them recognizable, whatever the historical period. The cardinal symptoms of the psychosis, depression and anguish that have been described since antiquity are largely identical today except for cultural differences. Generally speaking, where «normal» refers to an almost infinite and adaptable range of mental and biological human manifestations, «pathological» refers to a lessening – in terms of quantity and combinations – of the elements in this range. Art, on the contrary, like any creative process, proposes new answers that are added to the whole, even though colossal, of pre-existing possibilities. Thus, madness and art, which belong to different epistemological fields, are also opposed in terms of how they relate to reality (the fixedness and impoverishment of the disorder versus the novelty of creation). In addition, they illustrate an opposite relationship to humanness (alienation versus greater freedom). It is therefore most often not legitimate to explain one by the other in a linear fashion.

Thus, the power, the control, the interior solidity necessary for artists to accomplish their creation, and this while moving away from the references common to the social group to which they belong, are incompatible with the attack on volition, judgment and continuity characteristic of psychopathological states. Artists are therefore not mentally-ill individuals who are «healed» or «saved» by art, no more than mentally-ill individuals are artists through the simple fact of their disorder.

The second objection criticizes an excessively simplistic descriptive approach to psychopathology through art. It is indeed usually considered that some works of art obviously, almost automatically reflect aspects of psychiatric clinical observation. They are consequently considered as emblematic of certain semeiological aspects. Thus, Munch's *The Scream*, Dürer's *Melancholia*, the melancholic woman of Picasso's Blue Period or Goya's Black Paintings all conjure up – collectively and unequivocally – anguish and sadness. If we observe the artistic mechanisms at work, we soon perceive that artists achieve this effect, this illusion by staging their subject. This is especially obvious for musicians who, to express despair, anguish or the euphoria of love resort to a resonant production that transforms sadness into pathos and euphoria into jubilation. According to this analysis, a work of art stages one of the partial invariants of a psychopathological disorder (for instance, a scream in the case of anguish). This invariant, pushed to its paroxysm – and represented outside of the context in which it occurs – is acutely generalized. Singly, it becomes and sums up the disorder itself, when in reality it represents no more than the exaggeration of one of its partial features. This perspective is interesting but remains foreign to patients, distant from their subjectivity.

Describing the bipolar disorder: a twofold approach

The variety of manifestations – behavioural, emotional or cognitive – in patients suffering from bipolar disorder has driven clinicians to identify invariant manifestations, those that are both identified in the majority of the patients (specificity) and identifiable by different observers (interjudge reliability). They have organised the description of the disorder within a classification (nosography). This latter aspires not only to gather a number of different manifestations within a single pathological entity, but also to lay the foundations for teaching – clinical, certainly, but also explanatory and therapeutic teaching. When the purpose is all at once to describe, to explain and to teach the pathology, language and writing, i.e. words, are the most effective mediators. This is why every day, new books and new courses perpetuate and refine the medical knowledge on bipolar pathology. If, however, we maintain a concern for scientific rigor, we have to acknowledge that the nosographic method described above contains two major flaws. On the one hand, it does not account precisely for a whole series of clinical manifestations that are difficult to restore through language. Indeed, this latter, because of its temporal additive nature – by sequencing words one after the other – enables no more than the successive enunciation of the phenomena it is describing. Most mental phenomena, however, are concomitant and contradictory, calling upon mixed temporalities. Let us take the example of the feeling of pointlessness felt by the depressed patient at a given moment. This feeling appears for patients in a context of very complex concomitant representations: the disillusioned world that they perceive around them interpenetrates the idealized world of their past; the other humans who surround them appear to them as desirable, inaccessible, too intrusive and dangerous, all at the same time; they themselves see despair, the hope of returning to the ideal world, self-accusation and the feeling of being a victim as interweaving. Depressed patients therefore experience in a same moment of time an emotional mixture that cannot be understood as the immediate result of the mere addition of elements expressed in a verbal description. Clinicians must draw upon their own subjectivity to combine these elements and shape for themselves a representation of the mental world in which the patients live. On the other hand, in its attempt to be generalisable, description according to the smallest common denominator of symptoms such as those proposed in this nosography wipes out the singularity of the patient's experience, which in fact is also the manifestation of some of the invariant features of the disorder. Thus, jubilation and the impression of fundamental pointlessness, although subjective, are also perfectly characteristic of mania and depression respectively. To conceive and to teach these dimensions of subjectivity require mediators that will make them intelligible with precision but also without constraining them in their range of expression. Words, which as we have seen are perfectly adapted to the analytical description of phenomena, prove to be limited when they need to express and transmit the subjectivity to which we are referring. This is why, as we explained above, our choice went to the artistic mediator.

Subjectivity? Which subjectivity?
Our purpose is not to try to express the infinity of subjective states in the bipolar patient, but to identify «subjective invariants» in patients suffering from bipolar disorder with the purpose of describing them and attempting to organize them. We would like, for instance, to make the complex but characteristic dimensions of the bipolar disorder comprehensible to the clinician, such as thymic instability, certain characteristic emotional and cognitive mental processes, as well as alteration in the perception of time, of space and of other people. We would like to make it possible to understand, for instance, a characteristic procedure in manic patients' subjective perception of the world: that, for example, in which they conceive themselves as being an intimate part of an infinite whole, with which they feel they are in fusion and in harmony, thanks to which they have the intuition to reach universal order. Similarly, we would also like to be able to account for melancholic patients' painful subjective perception of a world where they see themselves as alone, outside of time and at the same time painfully condemned in the present.

The reader: subjectivity at work
Another advantage of this approach results from the fact that it is not closed, i.e., limited to the authors' impressions or opinions. We feel that using works of art as explanatory mediators of certain clinical dimensions of bipolar disorder is remarkably educational insofar as comprehension of the message plays out within the subjectivity of the reader. Our intention – indeed an ambitious one – is to make a number of universal constituents of bipolar disorder conceivable while accounting for the uniqueness of the patient's private experience, but letting our readers draw from their personal imagination to grasp it.

We can hope that patients, thus better comprehended, will become true protagonists in the care they are afforded.

PHILIPPE NUSS

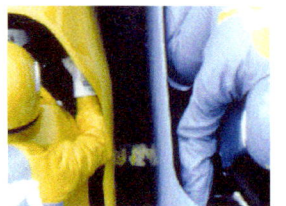

On the granite race track of the Isle of Man, two motorcycles with integrated sidecars prepare to start the race, side by side. One of the bikes is blue, the other yellow. The drivers are nailed to their handlebars, the team members ready to push with all their strength. The start is imminent, the determination extreme. Strangely, however, the two teams are running in opposite directions; besides, they seem to be ignoring one another, concentrated only on their individual determination. The same helicoidal logo, made of three bent legs as if in a perpetual race, is printed on all the runners' jumpsuits and on their engines. Could they all belong to the same team?

In bipolar-disorder observation, patients often describe the two pathological states, mania and depression, as opposite in terms of mood, of course, but similar in their determination, in the way they are triggered so abruptly; similar states, but seeming foreign to one another. When they are caught in either side of the disorder, bipolar patients describe themselves as trapped in an inexorable process that goes out of control and cuts them off from the world. What is experienced during these episodes is thus at the same time very strong and disconnected from ordinary perception. For this reason, the mood episode, the manic one in particular, despite its very serious consequences, seems not to have left any marks once the patient has recovered his health, so much does it strike him as belonging to another nature. This would imply, for the patient, that taking medication between the episodes of the disorder is not necessary, the two states having been experienced as parentheses, from which there would be nothing to learn. Treatment then appears all the more unnecessary that remission is felt as being permanent. And yet, a relapse is always possible: the opposite cycles are ever prepared to take a fresh start for a new race.

1994 Matthew Barney
Cremaster 4

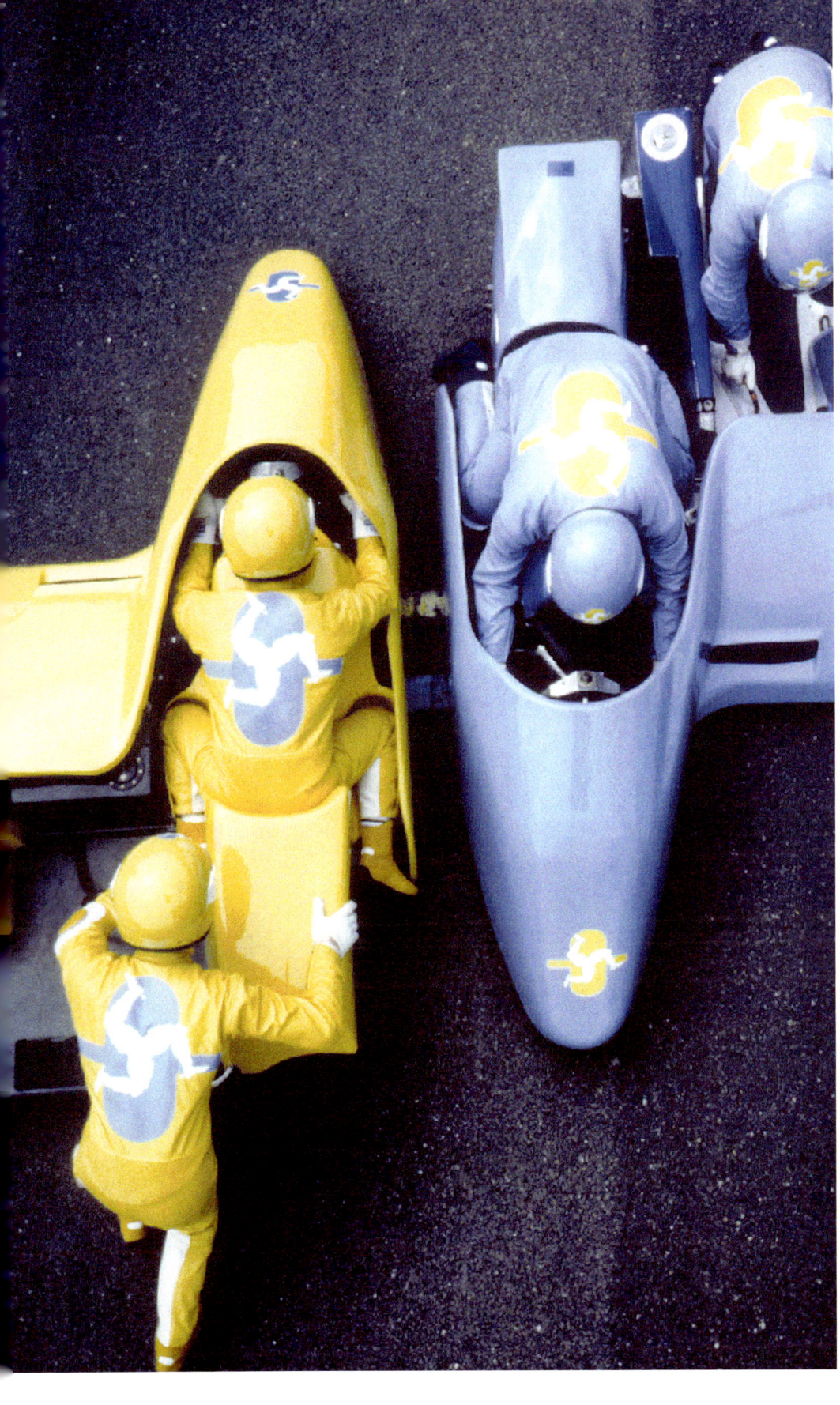

*Born in San Francisco in 1967, **Matthew Barney** first made his living as a doctor, a football player and a model. In 1991, he created his first Body Art performances in New York. It would take him eight years to compose his major work, a kind of contemporary fable or allegory in three dimensions, five films, and innumerable characters, installations and object sculptures, which he called Cremaster, the name of the testicular muscle that contracts in fear or in coldness. It is man's instant of indecision, placed between desiring something and fulfilling that desire, that fascinates Matthew Barney. His baroque staging masterfully and theatrically illustrates the human tragedy of an individual constantly torn between two opposite currents. The themes of ascension and descent confront each other in an inexorable succession.*

8

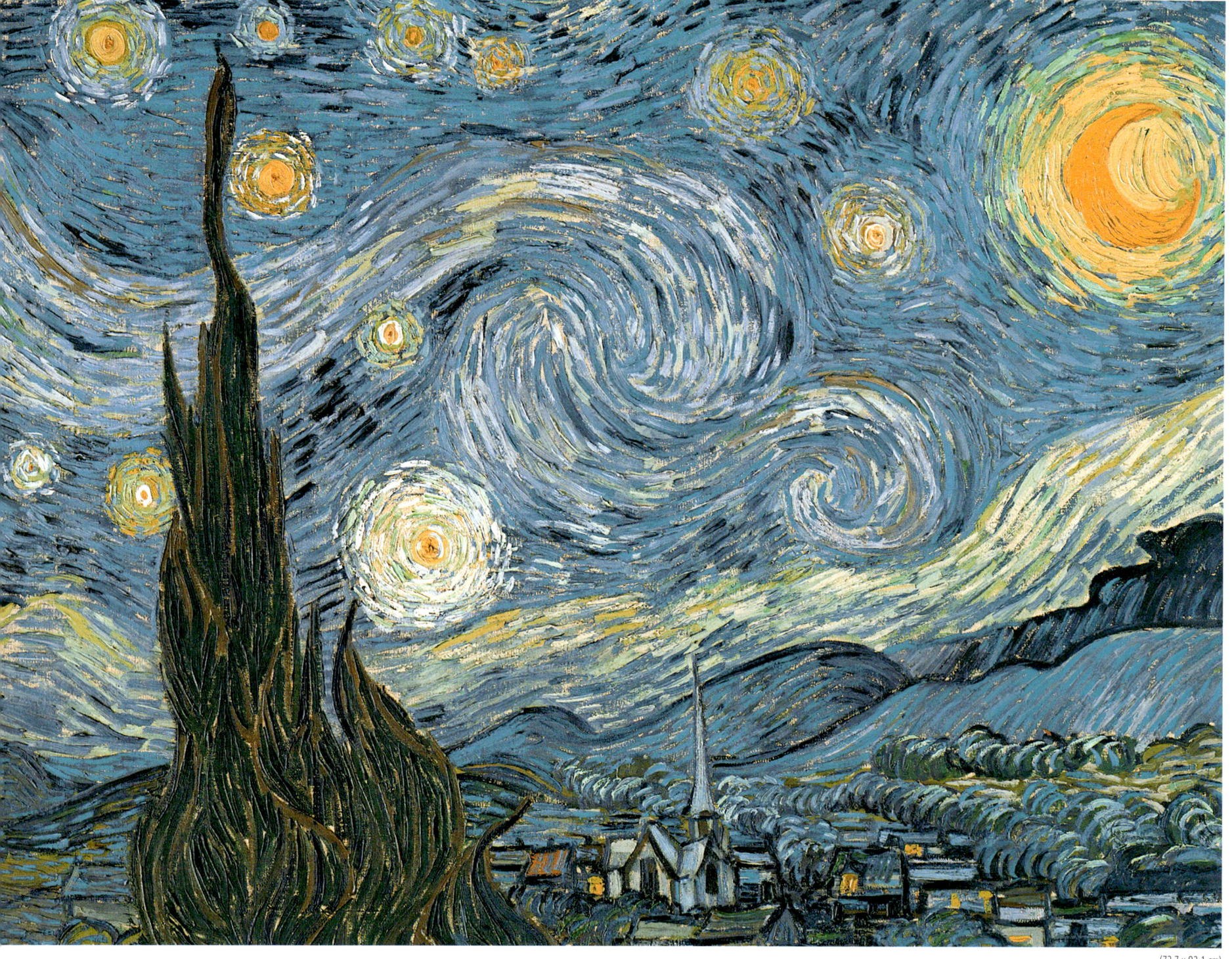

(73.7 x 92.1 cm)

LLUCINATION — TENSION — DISQUIETING STRANGENESS— HALLUCINATION — TENSION — DISQUIETING STRANGENESS—

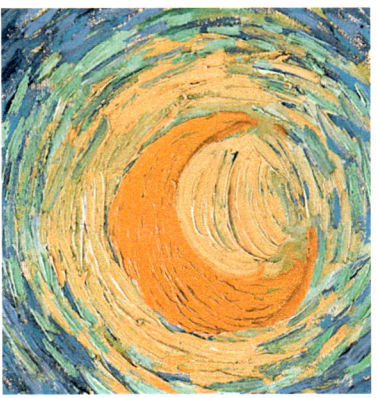

The immensity of the sky and the moving presence of suspended constellations immediately fill our visual field. The constellations abound, whirl and occupy the space with their warm presence. Below, the village, snuggled into the countryside, dozes in the darkness. In the foreground, the dark mass of a torch-like cypress connects the two parallel worlds, the land and the sky, and invites us to take part, as privileged witnesses, in the extraordinary dance of the universe. Once our amazement has vanished, we can see the detail of the curves of the clouds caught in the thick paste of the paint, the astounding lunar sun and the stream of light hugging the outline of the mountains on the horizon.

Similarly, the hallucinatory experience of the bipolar patient blends the familiar with the mysterious. This coexistence submits those who experience it to a twofold tension: experiencing the world such as it is and such as it is changed by hallucinations. As spellbound by the strangeness of what they experience as they are worried by the changes that they perceive in reality, patients have the feeling that they are taking part in an exceptional happening that reveals the unique nature of their experience. The real world appears to them then somewhat as the sleepy village of van Gogh's painting, distant and not very attractive. Solicited by these two experiences, they can either stop moving, as if hypnotised, or attempt to introduce the supernatural dimension into their familiar reality through some sort of action.

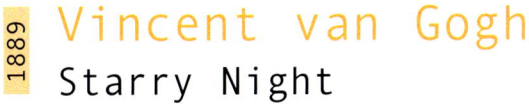

Vincent van Gogh
1889 Starry Night

*Son of a Dutch minister, **Vincent van Gogh** (1853-1890) worked with an art merchant then as a preacher in Belgium before devoting himself to painting. In eight years, from 1882 to his death, he produced close to eight hundred paintings, none of which was he able to sell. After his first dark and intimist paintings, his art became very colourful, coinciding with his discovery of the south of France. Settled in Arles, he convinced Gauguin to join him as he wished to work with him, but their joint plan did not work out. After having cut off his ear, he was hospitalised several times until he decided to settle in the asylum of Saint-Rémy, where he began painting again in large pasty strokes with the sinuous and turbulent touch that was his trademark. The last two months of his life, in Auvers-sur-Oise under the protection of Doctor Gachet, were a period of intense creation. But his illness left him but a short respite and, at age 37 on 27 July 1890, he shot a bullet though his chest.*

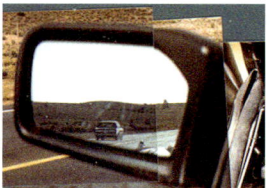

The photo collage positions us at the wheel of a luxury sports car. We are in the driver's seat. The dashboard in front of us seems to be reconstituted, like a puzzle of juxtaposed and sometimes mixed fragments of slightly different photos of the same passenger cell. Only its most significant details are unequivocally present in our visual field. We instinctively add the missing or unlikely parts of the montage as if we wished to restore the unity and the verisimilitude of the image and the place. This is first the case for the steering wheel, which, though truncated, we see as ready to be grasped. The Mercedes logo then comes to reassure us in our mental restitution work: a Mercedes cannot fail in its reputation. The circular, assuring instruments bring speed as well as dependability to mind: the machine is under control, all of its signals are reassuring, we can continue at a quick pace. The impression of speed is emphasised by the flash of light reflected on the steering wheel, illuminating its surroundings: it's a beautiful day, the road is wide open and we're speeding. No particular precaution then seems necessary. The driver's left foot, set firmly on the floor where the clutch should be, contributes paradoxically to the impression of speed at the same time that it determines the solidity of our position. Under the round speedometer in the frame of the steering wheel, an unlikely array of instruments, with familiar though incomprehensible outlines, is arranged around a sort of winged battery, incongruous but almost decorative. On our left, the door handle sparkles. Despite its obvious familiarity, we ask ourselves fleetingly: Could we open it if necessary? The wing mirror reminds us almost anecdotally that we are not alone on the road. Placed in an unlikely position, it appears as detached from the car, inaccessible and above all useless to the driver, who seems therefore to be able to do without it.

And by the way, where is this driver going so fast? Two photos of the road, almost perfectly adjusted, represent, much farther than the perspective might allow, a motorway worming peacefully into the nearly desert Arizona landscape. Except that in fact, the car is no longer on the road, but already on the verge: the road sign signalling a mythical Grand Canyon landscape seems to have attracted the driver more than the road that leads to it.

Reality as seen by manic patients is experienced as if it had been recomposed. Assailed by the multitude of stimuli that the world they perceive is made of, required to manage the pace and sequence of these stimuli, manic patients must in fact recompose their environment to be able to assimilate it. They need to select some parts over others and fill in the missing ones with close and plausible fragments in order to rebuild a single representation of the present as well as a coherent grasp of themselves. Despite this approximate reconstruction process, when a manic patient presents himself to us, the conviction in his tone and his presence incite us to believe him. We follow his lead and attempt to fill in his lack of coherence and unity: the beauty and the staging of the story incite us to believe it. As soon as we stand back from the patient's words or behaviour, we can in fact measure their improbability. The feeling of power and speed characteristic of the manic state give the patient a high, and a deep and immediate feeling of self-assurance, where a simple analysis of reality should on the contrary prompt him to caution. He believes to be safe from danger and does not hesitate to remove others from his landscape when they are not part of his enthusiastic project. Frequently on the edge of the road when they believe they are right in the middle of it, manic patients are often absorbed by the awesome landscape to which they aspire and they disregard the road that leads to it. Unfortunately, they sometimes drive on the verge and they are in danger of falling at any moment.

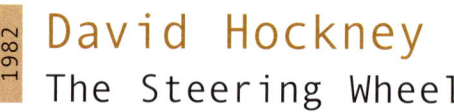

1982 — David Hockney — The Steering Wheel

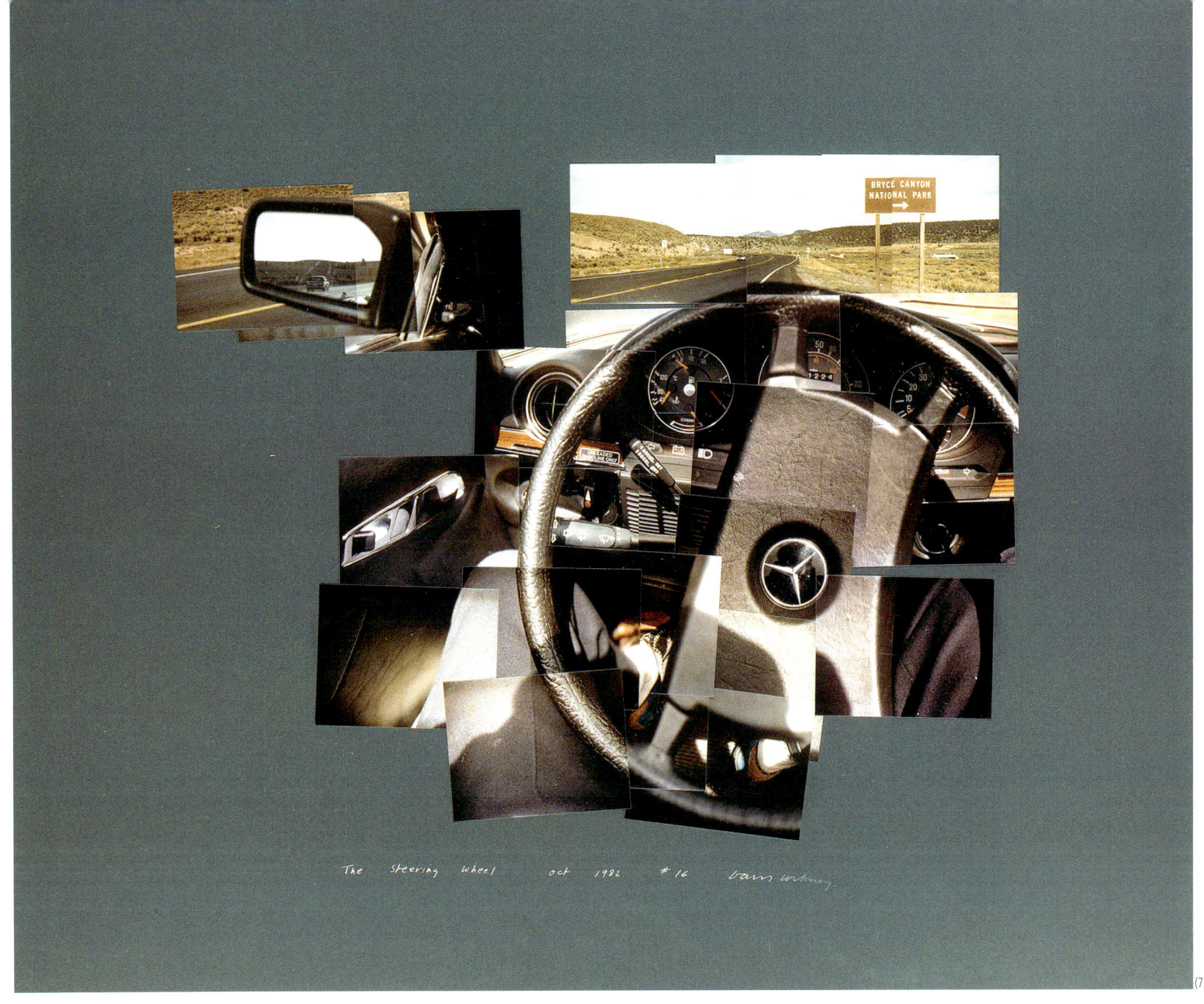

(75 x 91 cm)

Born in Great Britain in 1937 and a graduate of London's Royal College of Art, **David Hockney** has lived in California since 1963. Refusing all classification, he handles and re-interprets Pop Art, as well as abstraction or figuration, or even hyperrealism, with brio, producing portraits, landscapes and perspectives with painting, photography or collages… The recomposed realism of his collages, as well as the all-too-perfect vision of his ideal swimming pools in tart colours under the California sun represent a paradoxical reality made of obvious simplicity and ease while at the same time they are the reflection of solitude. Thus, despite a visual world that looks like it is made of Hollywood sets, David Hockney is in love with truth. He opens up, and depicts his desires just as he does the homosexuality that he wishes, he says, to assume with a minimum of honesty. Does he want to remind us that reality is elsewhere, beyond the appearances of things and people?

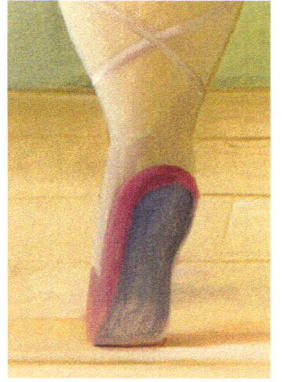

The grand battement a la seconde that Botero's ballerina executes with her back to the bar is both impeccable and pathetic. Her leg is indeed perfectly raised, her hip is low – we can see the sole of her ballet shoe – her hand en couronne is just above her forehead, her other hand is resting lightly on the bar. And yet, even more than the dancer's opulent shapes, her lower back packed into one piece, her motionless face and her eyes gazing forlornly upward convey a feeling of heaviness and fixedness. The impression produced by her tutu grown too short, along with her breasts badly contained in her tunic, is more an impression of childhood nostalgia than grotesque. The almost amateurish central framing of the dancer at the bar is disturbing, because the performance itself occupies the entire canvas with no apparent art, in a sort of pathetic turgidity. Although the entire canvas is occupied by the dancer, she herself seems no more there for the viewer than for the Dance.

The grand battement a la seconde, dancing on points and ballet in general are usually associated with joy, accomplishment, youth and elation in dance technique. Botero's ballerina conjures up stoical solitude instead. The outer form of what usually and almost automatically suggests youth and accomplishment is well represented: a perfectly controlled technique and a rose in the middle of the forehead. It has, however, the opposite effect. What we see is a canonical form, graceless and embarrassing. Manic patients often resort, in their clothing and gestures, to archetypal demonstrations of happiness (laughter and cheer, excessive movements, eccentric clothes that are over-determined in their significance). What often makes this behaviour so surprising, or even both laughable and wretched, is its inappropriateness to the context. More than abnormal, a manic patient's behaviour is ill-timed or out of place, it is inopportune. It is frankly unbecoming, that is, in conflict with the conventions of the moment and the place. As for this ballerina, what we perceive in the manic patient, blended into the excessiveness of the performance, is a part of sadness, or even of despair. In some cases, the presence of these two emotional states is obvious and simultaneous. This state of labile emotional moods is called a mixed state or dysphoric mania.

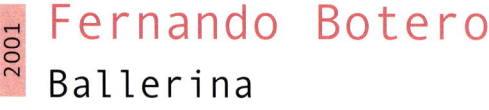

2001 **Fernando Botero**
Ballerina

Fernando Botero *was born in Medellín, Colombia, in 1932. After having won a painting prize as a young man in Bogotá, he started out for Europe and stayed in Barcelona, Madrid and Florence, where he developed a passion for Renaissance art. Categorically turning his back on abstraction, he began to paint work of generous volume as early as 1956. Indeed, Botero's trademark is plumpness. He sees the world as swollen, bloated and puffed up, which he reflects in a very personal form of mannerism blending influences of the Renaissance and of pre-Columbian art. "When I deform things," he says, " I enter a subconscious world rich in folk images." For Botero, art is, above all, distortion. He denies that he paints fat persons. He creates full and abundant forms. A true humanist, he is the author of a flourishing human comedy where all the world's actors are pinned into derisory or grandiose scenes of family, civilian or military life. He has exposed in the world's greatest Museums as well as in Paris for a remarkable retrospective of his sculptures on the Champs Elysées.*

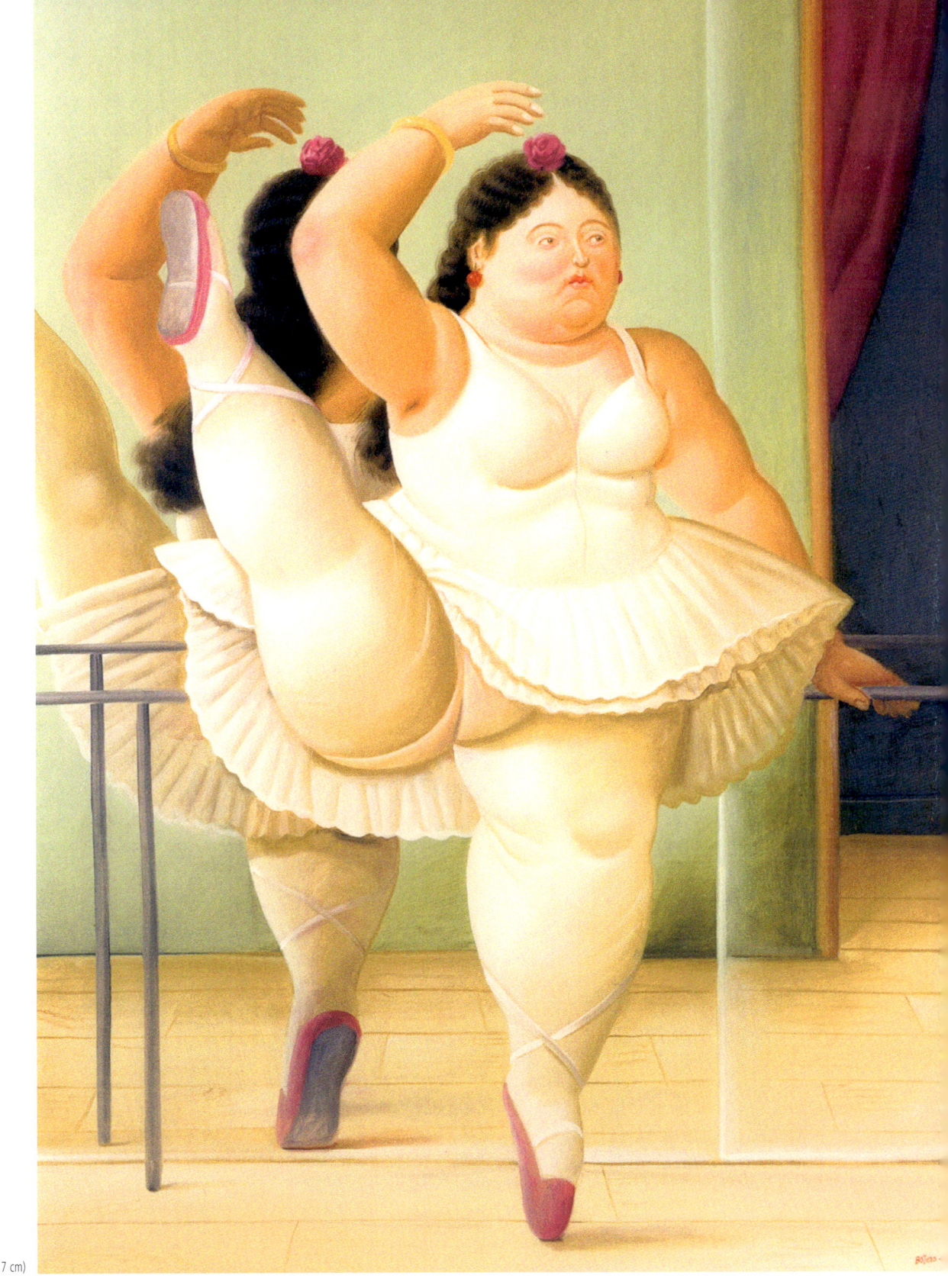

(309.9 x 386.7 cm)

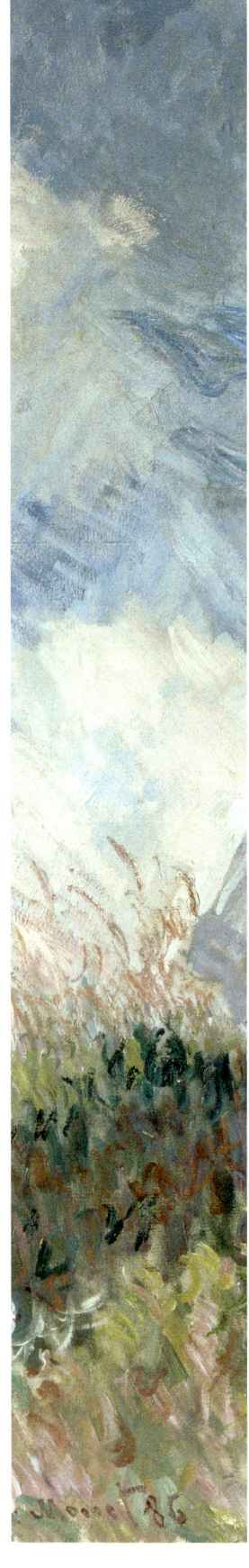

This pale-coloured woman's silhouette, barely distinct from an uncertain sky, appears to us as if we were lying in the grass and watching her without her being aware of us. She seems absolutely alone in the vastness of a Nature that absorbs her entirely and draws her to the point of vanishing into a whirlwind of moving clouds. In the shade, her right arm, the one holding the parasol, is in contrast with the rest of the painting made entirely of luminous strokes. The only dark point of the work, it allows, by contrast, the light and the air to gather the figure and the natural surroundings into an immaterial whole, ready to spin or perhaps vanish like a dream. The apparition, whose face can hardly be made out through a thin veil, is in unison with the landscape that surrounds it. A dreamer in the heart of a dream, she lets her thoughts wander like clouds in the wind and it is precisely her absence that makes her so present to us.

Solitude, like pain, is an experience full of contradictions. The sadness, the feeling of pointlessness of patients who are depressed and their impression of inability, obviously stir up their impression that they are alone. The fugitive ideas, the instability and the loss of control of the manic patient's mood reflect another form of solitude: that of the difficulty, or even the impossibility of communicating. In both cases, the solitude is born from an opposition: the opposition between the impression of nothingness of patients in a depressed state, who perceive the outside world as an organised unit where everything is purported to be easy, and the cup-runneth-over impression of patients in a manic state, who feel misunderstood and unable to be integrated into the society in which they live.

In contrast with this experience of absolute isolation, there is, as much in manic as in depressed persons, a sort of intuition that their state is the manifestation of a universal order, or disorder. One who is depressed perceives his solitude through a pessimistic analysis of life, life in a society with contemptible rules and obviously finite. Hence it seems legitimate to him to think that there is no possible solution because reality is truly hopeless. Thus, the world from which he feels fundamentally cut off is at the same time in unison with his solitude. For manic patients, the world's agitation, in its infinite, almost vertiginous variety, enters into resonance with what they feel and attests, as far as they are concerned, to the accuracy of their personal experience made of excess, movement and an infinity of interpretations. Paradoxically, the solitude of manic or depressive states is as much a manifestation of the subject's being cut off from his environment as an expression, according to the patient, of the fact that he is fully part of a universal order.

Thus, absolutely alone and in unison with creation at the same time, bipolar patients feel a form of existential contradiction in which they perceive themselves as living an experience, the uniqueness of which wounds as much as it affirms their existence.

Claude Monet
1886 — Woman with Umbrella Turned to the Left

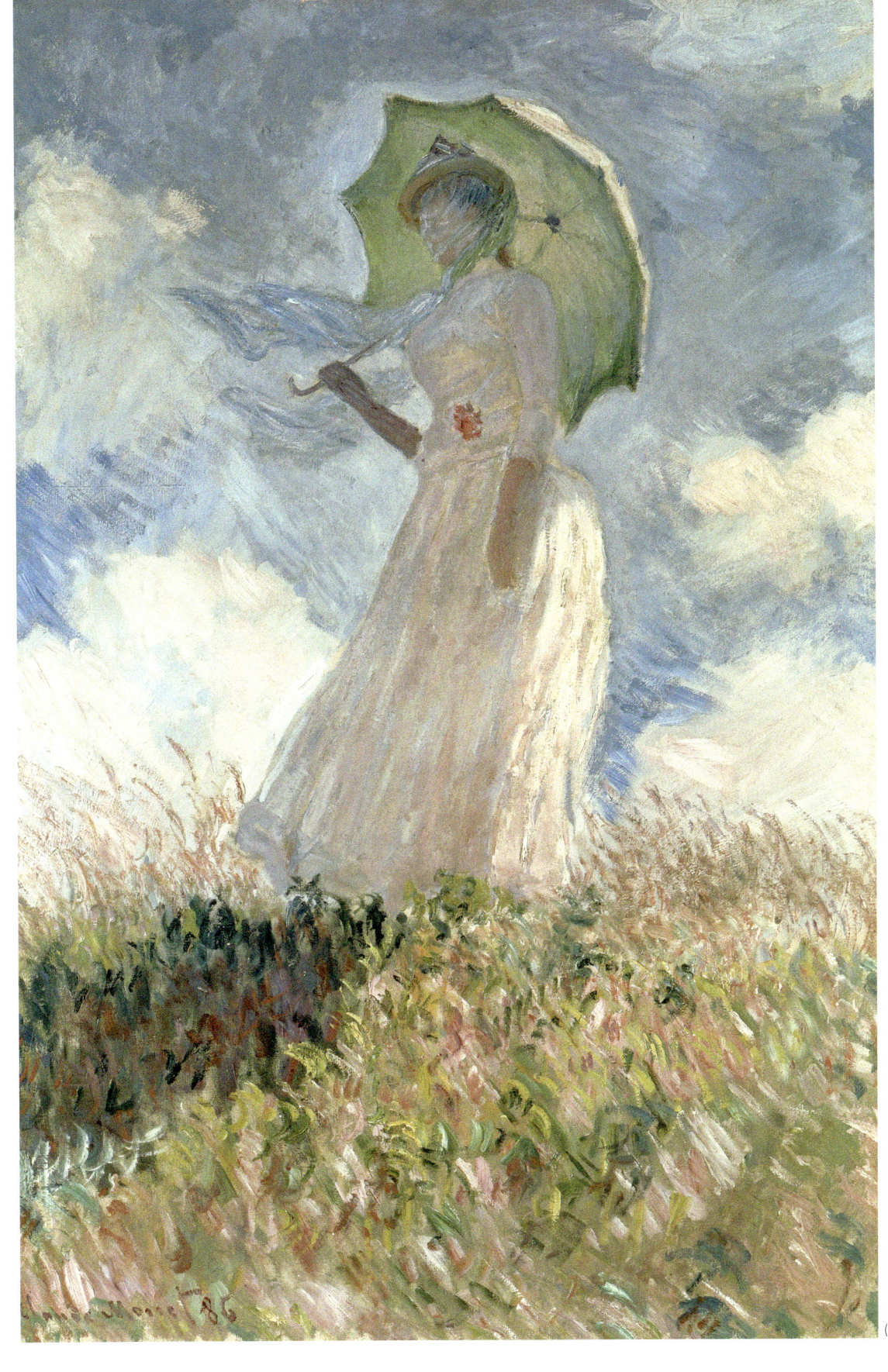

(88 x 131 cm)

This painting, also known as La femme à l'Ombrelle, *Woman with Umbrella, is an echo to another painting of the French artist* **Claude Monet** *(1840-1926), which shows Camille, his first wife, in Argenteuil in 1875. Here, however, his step-daughter Suzanne Hoschedé is given an even more aerial treatment, with no concern for resemblance. At that time, Monet was already painting practically nothing but landscapes. It was light, wind, and the elusive that fascinated the leading figure of the Impressionists.*

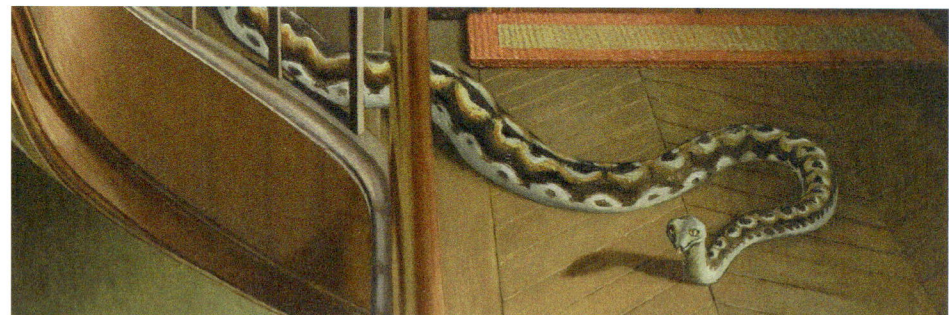

Pierre Roy
1927
Danger on the Stairs

This is a traditional stairwell in an bourgeois building. We climb up the well-waxed staircase, vaguely aware of the walls carefully painted in trompe-l'oeil. We reach a landing. Not a noise to be heard. No one. A closed door with polished brass knobs, with an impeccable doormat, is illuminated by the light from the window. We prepare to continue our climb. But an intruder is there and interferes: a silent snake, and it is staring at us. We can no longer go on. It is coming from above, perhaps from where we intended to go. Our solitude, which until that moment was associated with stillness, becomes agonizing: we are facing it alone. The beast will not turn back, we can see that. The only option is to flee. And then? Will it be possible to come back?

The spontaneous, unforeseeable and recurring nature of manic or depressive episodes induce in the patients an impression of existential insecurity. They know that the disorder can come up again at any moment. Yet they long for serenity and are prepared to make a lot of sacrifices to avoid another relapse. They dream of a space that is sure and safe from danger. This situation generates an ambivalence: the efforts that they are willing to make, tending towards this safety constantly remind them, at the same time, of their fragility. Even though their entire being rebels against the disorder, the threat or the suffering of a relapse makes them recoil: they will henceforth have to cope with the dis-quietude generated by the bipolar disorder.

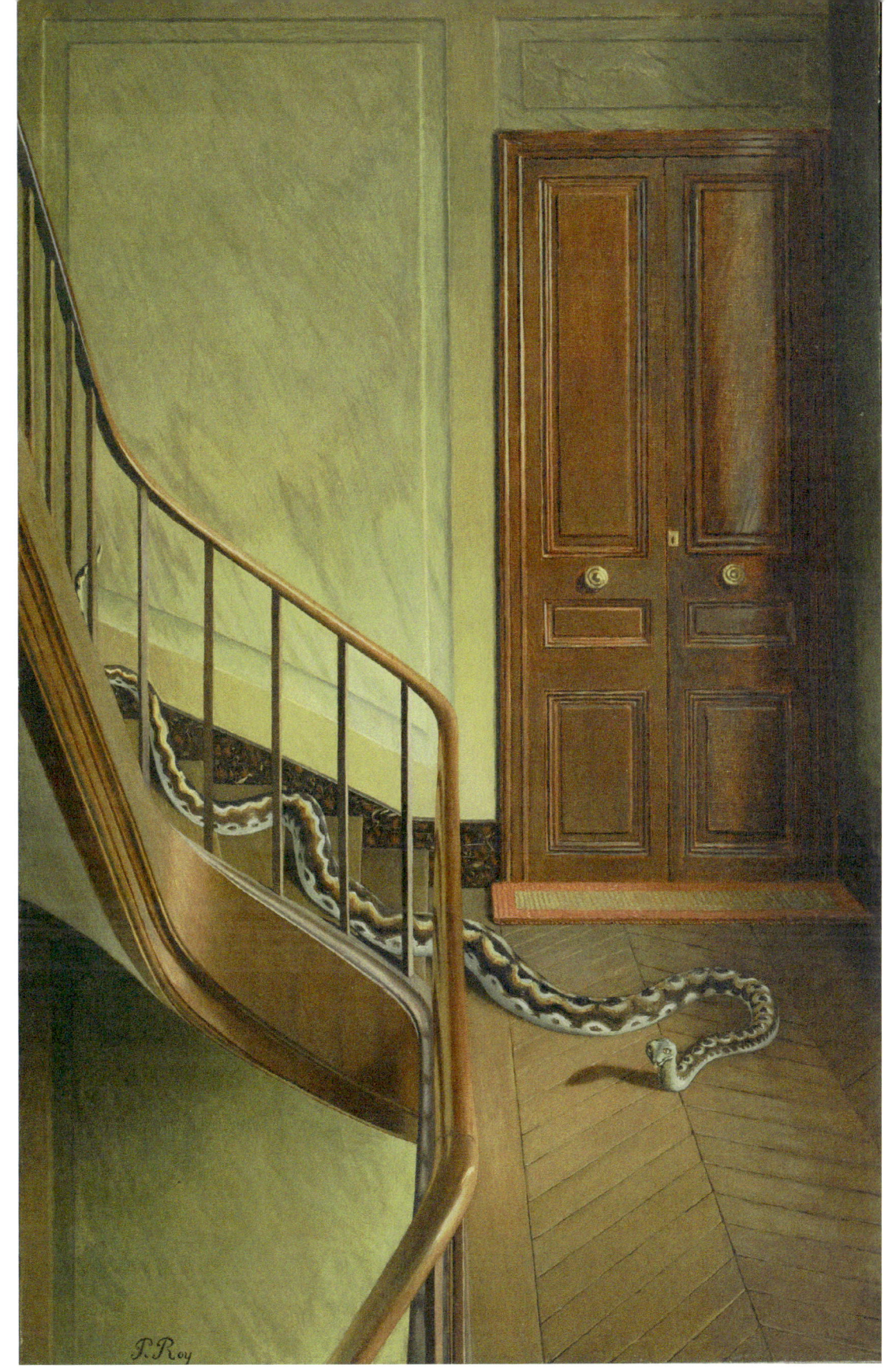

The work of **Pierre Roy** (1880-1950), painter-engraver from Nantes (France) and a friend of Guillaume Apollinaire, is part of the surrealist movement but remains profoundly free, original and unclassifiable. "As a painter, I have absolutely no philosophy," he would say. "Whenever I paint anything at all, I am completely abandoned to the pleasure of painting. I haven't the slightest intention of symbolism. But very often, sometimes long after I've finished my painting, I realise what has inspired me and what my painting means."

(91.4 x 60 cm)

—INSECURITY — AMBIVALENCE — RELAPSE —INSECURITY — AMBIVALENCE — RELAPSE —INSECURITY — AMBIVALENCE —

Bipolar Disorder in 1854: A Description

"Dual Form Insanity"

 There are no states which show more marked differences the one from the other and more striking contrasts than melancholia and mania.

The melancholic is weak, timid and irresolute; his life is spent in inertia and mutism; his conceptions are slow and confused.

The maniac, by contrast is full of confidence, of energy and audacity; he deploys the greatest activity, and his loquacity has no limits.

It would therefore seem, in theory, that two States so opposed must be foreign one to another, and that a great distance must separate them.

This is not, however, that which is demonstrated by observation. Indeed we see, in many cases, melancholia succeed mania, and vice versa, as if a secret bond united these two diseases.

These singular transformations have been often reported.

Pinel speaks of attacks of melancholia which degenerate into mania.

According to Esquirol, it is not unusual to see mania alternate, and in a very regular manner, with pulmonary phthisis, hypochondria and lypemania.

These alternations of melancholia and mania have also been observed by Mr Guislain, and I might add by almost all the authors; but although the fact is well-established, it seemed to me that it had not sufficiently been studied.

By bringing together and comparing a certain number of observations, it becomes clear that there exist quite numerous cases in which it is impossible to consider in isolation and as two distinct disorders the excitation and the depression which succeed each other in a single patient. This succession, indeed, is not a matter of chance, and I have been able to confirm that there exist connections between the duration and the intensity of the two states, which are clearly nothing other than two periods of a single attack. The consequence of this view is that these attacks properly belong neither to melancholia nor to mania, but that they constitute a special kind of mental alienation, characterised by the regular existence of two periods – one of excitation and the other of depression.

It is of this kind of madness which I shall try here to indicate the principal characteristics. I shall refer to it provisionally by the name dual form madness.

I believe I can do no better, in order to give an exact idea of the attacks, than to cite a few observations, restricting myself, moreover, to the details which shall seem to me the most important.

Observation I - Miss X., today aged twenty-eight years, had several attacks of mania from the age of sixteen to eighteen. After remaining in good health for three years, she experienced a relapse, and since then her illness has not ceased. This condition returns by attacks, of a duration of approximately one month.

During the first fifteen days, one observes all the symptoms of a profound melancholia; then all of a sudden the mania breaks forth and lasts for the same time.

When the period of depression begins, Miss X. feels herself prey to a sadness which she cannot overcome. A sort of a numbness little by little invades her entire being.

Her physionomy takes on an expression of suffering, her voice is weak, her movements of extreme slowness; soon the symptoms become worse, the patient remains immobile and mute on her chair; all effort becomes impossible, the slightest stimulation is painful, the light of day fatigues her. Miss X. is very well aware of what is happening around her; she understands the questions addressed to her, but replies slowly, in monosyllables, and in such a low voice that her words may be heard but incompletely. Together with all the symptoms above, there is insomnia, loss of appetite, constant constipation; the pulse is weak and slow.

After three or four days, the physionomy is already profoundly affected; the eyes are shadowed, sunken and without expression, the complexion pale and yellow.

When this state has endured fifteen days, it suddenly ceases during the night, and the general torpor is replaced by an exaltation of the greatest liveliness.

The following day, the patient is seen to be animated in her features, bright in her gaze, lively in her speech, her movements sudden and rapid; she is unable to remain one moment in the same place, and runs back and forth as if pulled by an irresistible force. Having been confused, her intelligence acquires vivacity. Miss X. would grasp with remarkable sagacity everything which, in the persons around her, might lend itself to ridicule. Her eloquence would be inexhaustible and express itself through continual epigrams. In this new state the insomnia would continue, but the appetite was restored. After fifteen days, calm would return almost suddenly. Miss X., who recalled everything she had said during the second period of her attack, would appear a little sad and confused; but soon she resumed her ordinary habits.

Unfortunately, the intermission would be of short duration; rarely has it lasted two or three months; usually, it is after fifteen or twenty days that a new attack breaks out.

The patient, who during the period of depression had taken only a wholly insufficient quantity of nourishment, would lose weight very rapidly. On one occasion, the loss was 12 pounds in fifteen days.

In the period of reaction and during the intermission, the appetite would be very great, and the increase in weight would also take place with great rapidity.

As for the moral and intellectual state of the patient during the two periods of the attack, I can give no better idea than by citing the following observation, in which the patient himself describes what he experienced.

Observation II - This madman, cured by Willis, had attacks similar in almost every way to those I have just described; only each period lasted ten days instead of fifteen.

"I would always await with impatience, says the patient, the attack of agitation which would last ten to twelve days, more or less, because I enjoyed throughout it a sort of beatitude: everything seemed easy to me; no obstacle could stop me in theory, nor even in reality; my memory suddenly acquired a singular perfection; I could remember long passages from the Latin authors. Ordinarily, I have difficulty in finding two rhymes at once, and yet at this time I would write in verse as rapidly as in prose; I was crafty and full of all kinds of expedients.

"The indulgence of those who, in order not to push me too far, allowed me to give free rein to all my fantasies reinforced in my mind the conviction of my superior powers and reinforced my audacity. My insensitivity to cold, to heat, to all the small inconveniences of life, further justified it. Finally, a profound and concentrated egoism made me relate everything to my person.

"However, he adds, if this first kind of illusion made me happy, I was only the more to be pitied in the state of despondency which always followed it, and which would last approximately as long. I regretted all my past actions, and even my very ideas. I was timid, ashamed, pusillanimous, incapable of action, whether physical, or moral. The change from one of these states to the other took place suddenly, with no transition, and almost always during sleep."

I could simply repeat the details above for the intellectual and moral state of the female patient whose observation I read earlier. In this case, I have preferred to report the words of the patient cured by Willis. […]

Jules Gabriel François Ballarger, 1895

Anthology of French Language Psychiatric Texts. Ed F.R. Cousin, J. Garrabé, P. Morozov. *Transl J Crisp, Les empêcheurs de penser en rond*, 1999.

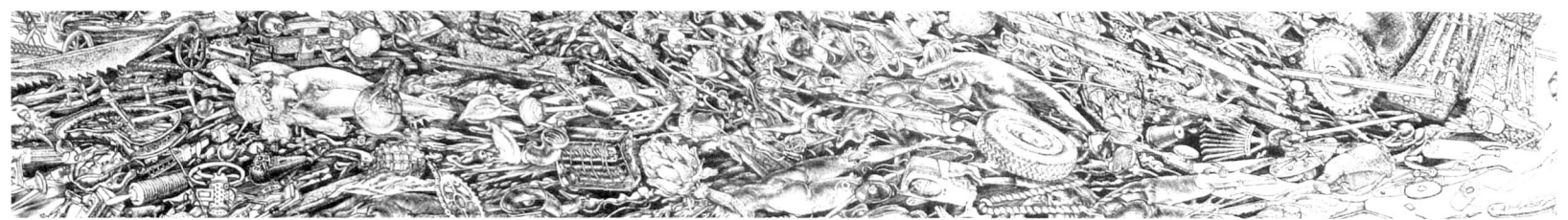

One's gaze is irresistibly drawn towards a vanishing point placed on the right of this engraving, in the direction of which converges, as if sucked up, a heterogeneous multitude. Only a beetle, in the foreground, can be immediately identified because it is larger than everything else. A meticulous examination of the composition of this vast sewage field haphazardly reveals: pieces of sheet metal, a helicopter, a hunting horn, a syringe, a domino, human or animal corpses on the drift… The objects here are mingled without any order; devitalised, they pile up like the waste of a plethoric world that will never be able to eliminate it. The drawing is done in extremely minute detail; the innumerable and elusive objects as a whole impose themselves with no transcendence, an impression made more powerful by the chisel technique used by the artist.

The melancholic patient features a relationship to death that can be illustrated by this work, "Un point c'est tout": "Period. Nothing More". Indeed, the death of which such patients speak to us and to which they say they aspire is the result, according to them, of an objectifying analysis of the inanity of the world's objects. These latter, populating – or even invading – their most immediate daily life, no longer appear to them as instruments at the service of their projects, but in their most immediate materiality, as perishable and forgotten after having been fleetingly used. The same is true for those who surround the melancholic patient: he feels fundamentally cut off from them. Indeed, the fact that each of us is autonomous inescapably leads to having a part of ourselves be unknowable by others. Thus, the diversity that is associated with the differences in human beings, far from being perceived as a source of wealth, is regarded by melancholic patients as being the testimony of their absolute isolation. In addition, and beyond this analysis deformed by the prism of depression, melancholic patients are driven in spite of themselves by an autonomous current that beyond them, leads to a point they call Death. The ideas of death perceived by the melancholic patient should thus also be understood as a symptom generated by the depression itself and not only as the consequence of a pessimistic analysis of the world. Thus, the death of which the melancholic patient speaks, contrary to the one that healthy persons can perceive, is completely deprived of transcendence.

Jean-Pierre Velly
1978
Period. Nothing More

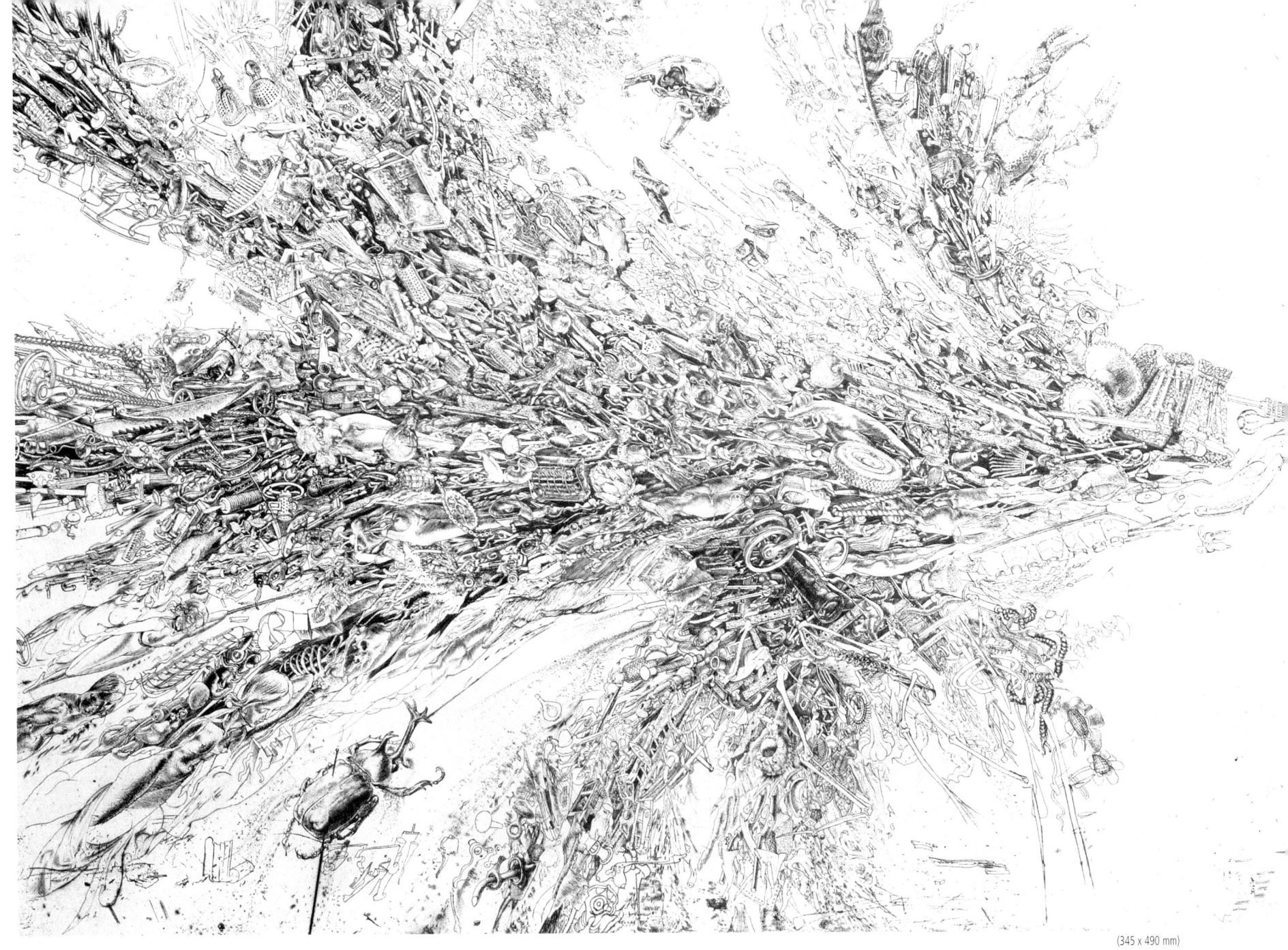

(345 x 490 mm)

*The engraver **Jean-Pierre Velly** (1943-1990) was Breton by birth and Italian by adoption. He enjoyed describing in extremely minute detail the contemporary world grappling with its pollution and humankind in distress fleeing what it has generated. It is as a drawing virtuoso that he chiselled his copper plates with a dry-point, making a whole universe emerge within just a few square inches.*

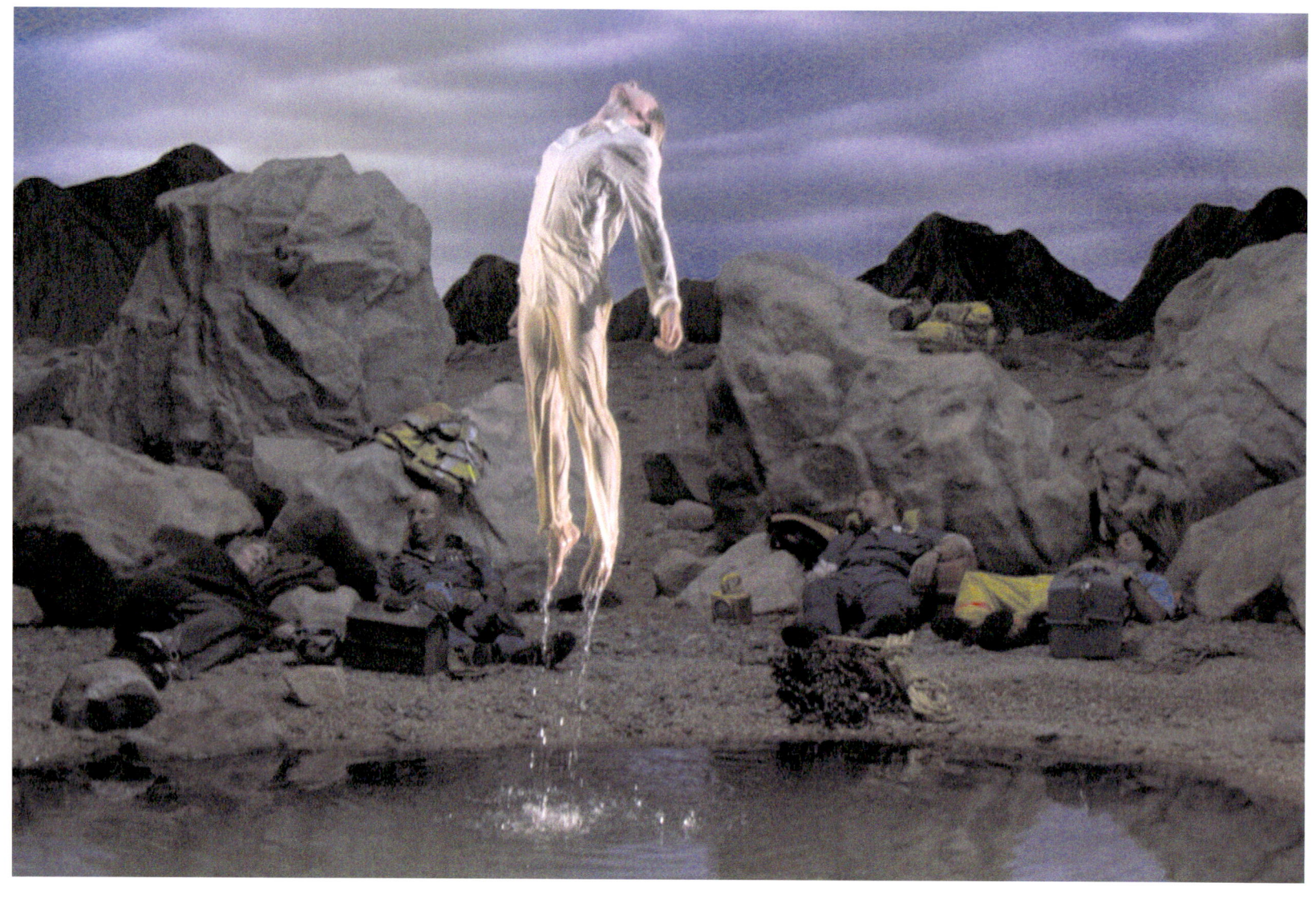

Bill Viola *was born in New York in 1951. He began doing research in video in 1972 after having studied art at New York University. His influences include John Cage's music, Godard's films and Beckett's plays (a man alone, crushed by the enormity of nature). A follower of eastern philosophies, he has tried to express the role of mental processes as projected into the perception of reality. Thinking must be greater than reality. In his video installation of 1976,* He Weeps for You, *a drop of water takes on a gigantic, almost cosmic dimension.*

To stage time, light and space, Viola uses slow motion like a microscope. He plays on rhythm, deceleration or acceleration, to give the images a mental character: for Viola, the place where the work truly exists is not in the image on the screen or the wall, but in the mind and heart of the person who views it. Underlying his work are the fundamental questions: the meaning of life, the human condition, the passage between life and death, the reason for the existence of human beings in the universe, and their relationship with the natural elements and the galaxy.

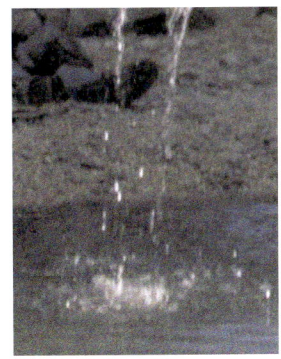

The light of dawn radiating into a blue and cloudy sky sheds an even luminosity on a mineral landscape made of large blocks of stone scattered on thick, drab sand. These harsh and inhospitable surroundings, almost lunar or desert-like, are mellowed by the presence of a small area of water in the foreground. Close to the water, four characters lying in a variety of positions are sleeping very deeply with their head against the rocks. It seems odd to see them gathered in this abandoned place. Three workers, still wearing their dungarees, their tool box close at hand, are resting from a technical or mining job, enigmatic in this desert-like world. The fourth sleeper, a traveller with greyish hair and clothes from another period, seems to have escaped from a stagecoach or a steam-powered train. The stillness and the depth of their sleep suggest that the previous day was tiring. Each of them seems to be caught up in his own history, his own dream. Suspended in the air in a vertical position, surprised while in full ascension, a young man with wet, light-coloured clothes seems to has just emerged from the water. His head in hyperextension to the back, his upper back arched and his arms slightly apart are in contrast with the verticality of the lower part of his body. His position suggests ascension as much as it does trance. Contrary to the other characters, he is not asleep; he seems to be borne by a supernatural phenomenon beyond his will. The bilateral lighting in which he is swathed has no relationship to the light of dawn bathing the rest of the scene: what comes to mind is the lighting of a theatre stage. This particular lighting on the ascending subject makes him actually seem to be a source of light. The extreme aesthetics of the colouring, the contrast in the matters as well as the strong symbolic valence of the objects and the characters bring to mind the ideal and the supernatural. The different plastic treatment of the characters who are sleeping and of the one that is rising seeks to underscore that the latter is taking part in an experience that is inaccessible to the others or that they are unaware of.

During manic states, but also sometimes during melancholic states, some patients can present delusional symptoms with a mystical content. In the first case, there is often a revelation or the conviction of being the singular receiver of a divine message. The jubilation and the sensation of being part of a total and exclusive experience is usually combined with the perception of the immensity of the responsibility inherent to such a solicitation. During melancholic states, of course, the delusion has no jubilation attached to it. Perceptions and interpretations of damnation, sin and eternal punishment reinforce the patients' conviction that their own life is pointless. In manic states, these mystical experiences are often intense and brief. Emotional states vary, depending on the patient. These can be a total experience such as a trance or the sudden, sometimes incredulous discovery that their body or their close surroundings carry the unquestionable marks of a divine message intended for them. The themes vary according to the patient's culture and possible religious affiliation. We often observe, in the same patient, a mixture of references drawing from several religions or mythological themes. The messianic dimension is quite rare: the manic patient, invaded by a mystical delusion, does not seek to make others embrace his beliefs. This is understandable insofar as patients in a manic state are incapable of adjusting to their fellow beings. The mystical experiences of manic states are hence distinct from those of believers, whatever their faith, insofar as the latter's occur as part of a religion, i.e., etymologically speaking, that which binds.

Bill Viola
2002
Going Forth By Day, "First Light"

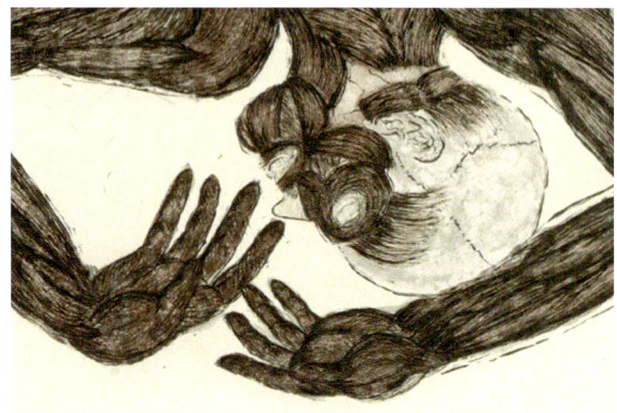

1992 **Kiki Smith**
Dream

On a sand- or eggshell-coloured background, an écorché (a human anatomical figure) is curled up as if he had been run aground. Behind the fragile protection of his arms, his body is the object of an insidious transformation. His abdomen grows heavy and his torso longer, and his arms are progressively dislocated while his legs wither away – there is no possible resistance. His white head alone, as if mummified, seems preserved from this upheaval. And yet this écorché is alive. The animal density of his contracted muscle masses does not suggest death.

A thin edging surrounds the figure's anatomical shape and shows what is happening inside, as if suffering could be X-rayed. We thus enter in spite of ourselves a space at the confines of birth and death, a primeval space that it is usually forbidden to see. A first reflex of shrinking back from this disclosure is immediately followed by the empathy that we can feel for the figure lying there. Struggling with these two visions that impose themselves with equal force, our almost embarrassed gaze hesitates with our concern for this dark mass, all at the same time a foetus and in the throes of agony, an animal and a humanoid.

We usually use the term of pain when speaking of physical suffering. The patients' great lesson is that mental disorder is painful too. They even describe it as more painful, as intolerable, beyond anything that they have felt before that. The expression "mental pain" is the one that they believe is closest to what they feel. "Mental" is not understood here in its mere sense of a good or bad mental condition. Mental pain does not exclusively qualify depression or sadness, it also qualifies a way of being in the world that is inherent to the disorder. What physical pain and mental pain have in common is that they burden the mind and annihilate thought, that they make the present far too present and the moment impossible to inhabit. In addition, however, mental pain induces self-dispossession. Like the figure slowly transforming itself behind the pathetic protection of its arms, ailing subjects feel powerless to live their own life and watch, alarmed and lost, the transformation of their intimate being. Being both the object and the viewer of the upheavals caused by the disorder, patients in an acute phase – and this is what they will never wish to experience again – suffer from the nightmare that their life has become, as much as from their inability to organise what they perceive of it. They are thus twice abandoned, by the world and by themselves.

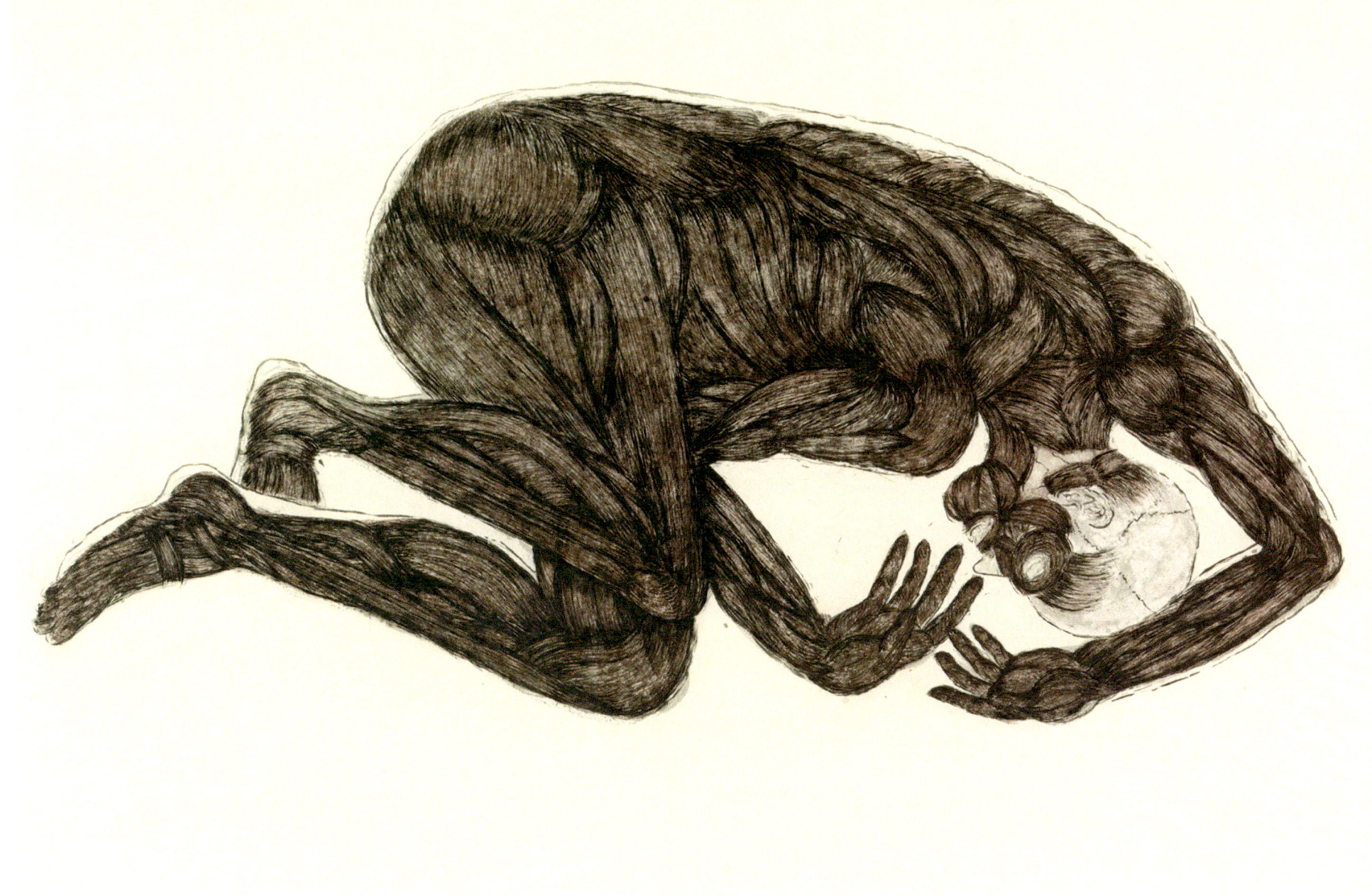

(106.2 x 195.8 cm)

Kiki Smith was born in Nuremberg, Germany, in 1954 and has lived in New York since 1976. The subject of all her engravings, sculptures, drawings and photographs is the body, human or animal, the pivotal theme of her work and a metaphor of the world. Conceived as a transient space between the outside and the profound self, she perceives the body as a universal resonance chamber and the centre of one's singularity. In her representation of it she associates outside appearance and the depiction of inner organic functions by which she is fascinated. Without any grandiloquence, she attempts to approach the being in its finiteness and its fragility, pursuing thus over the years her thinking on human nature assorted with a quest of self.

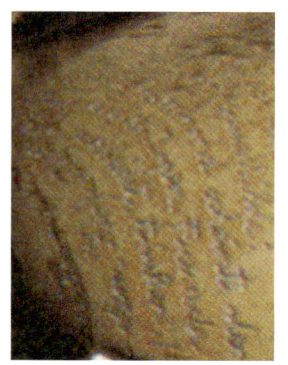

The polished pebble, well-protected in its shell, hardly seems to be made of porcelain. Its grain is soft, it almost seems to have animal flesh, it radiates a peaceful light: it is in its place, here, like a mountain in a landscape. We wish to come closer to it, but not to take it. We would like to touch it, but not to move it. The polish of its uncovered surface calls to be caressed. The delicate granite of its written side has the authority of secret, sacred texts. The opening of the shell imposes silence. Whose is the hand that gently detached a fragment of the shell and laid it right next to it? It matters not how and why it has been broken since at any moment the fragile envelope can be closed again.

During acute episodes, whether manic or depressive, the first step of the treatment is said to be "curative", which means that it tackles in the illness the disorder, which it attempts to reorganise as closely as possible to the usual behaviour of the subject. The disorder of the illness constitutes, in fact, an organisation of sufficiently stable symptoms, since all patients suffering from this disorder, all over the world, express this "disorder" in a recognizable way. Treating the acute episode therefore consists in going from one order to another, from that of the illness to that of health. The difference between these two orders is that that of the illness constrains the patient while that of health is associated with a high degree of freedom. In bipolar disorder, there persists, once the episode is healed, a fragility inherent to the illness: the danger of a relapse is indeed part of the nature of the disorder. The second stage of the treatment therefore consists in preventing this vulnerability from moving into a new episode. The status of the treatment then changes. After being curative, it becomes preventive. And quite often, the same medication can fulfil the two functions successively. Like this pebble in its broken shell, bipolar patients have not lost their profound unity during a pathological episode, even though in these moments their speech seems to be disorganised. On the other hand, the patients' vulnerability consists, if they do not protect themselves, in losing the protective shell that grants them the necessary distance in their relationship to the world. Made bare by the illness, they express their distress in two apparently opposite styles. The manic response can be understood as a reaction to the perception of reality with no filter to afford some distance; reality then flows in from all sides and sparkles with vitality for the patient, who believes he can easily manage the flood. The depressive response, for its part, could be associated with the perception by the patient of his extreme fragility: without his protective shell, he feels powerless to face the harsh presence of reality.

The treatment, in its preventive objective, must be seen as a deliberate action – i.e., non-constrained – of the patient. Everything happens as if taking his treatment consisted in delicately putting the shell that was opened during the pathological episode back in its initial position.

Linde Wächter-Lechner
Earth Song

1990

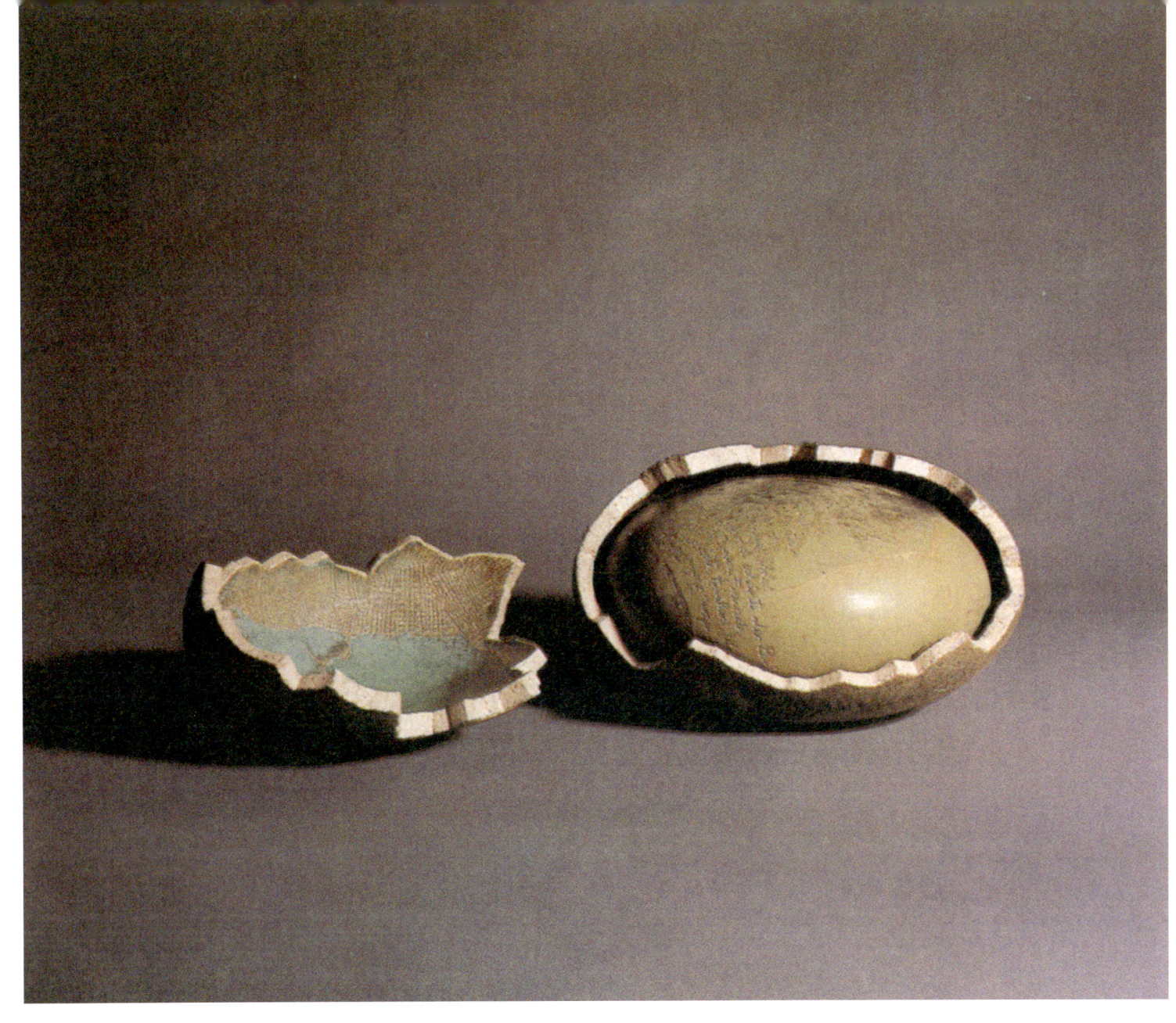

(195 x 100 x 31 cm)

Born in Austria in 1944, **Linde Wächter-Lechner** has lived and worked in France since 1976. Settled in France since 1976, she exposed her ceramics in the United States and in Europe. Her sensual approach to matter has the gift of transforming the inert into nearly living and allows her to explore a zone at the confines of the mineral, the plant and the animal worlds. The text that can be distinguished on the pebble of "Earth Song" is an excerpt of "Porcelain Pavilion" by the poet Li Po (701-762).

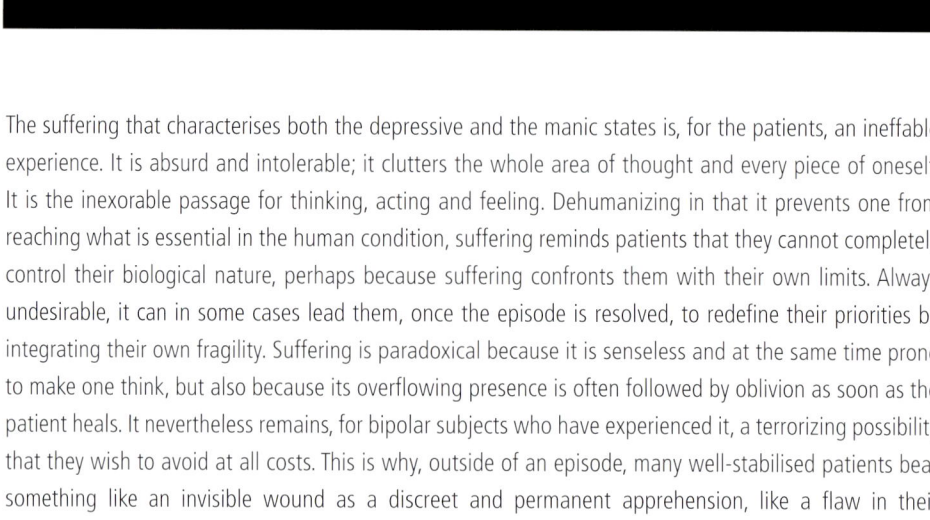

These two fragments of the Issenheim Altarpiece are as much the embodiment of the sufferer's arms as they evoke the knotted twining stems of a bloodless plant. The hands, with fingers torn apart into a corolla, are both a call and resignation. Although one sees nothing else, the entire subject is present and identified as the one who suffers. One, who in this detail, is not just Christ the person but any person suffering. The dead-wood treatment of the arms and the nearly living one of the badly squared crossbar call to mind the passage, in death, of the human status to that of an object of Nature, as well as the idea, dear to the Romantics, that Nature is in correspondence with men's suffering.

Matthias Grünewald
1512-1516
Issenheim Altarpiece
details

The suffering that characterises both the depressive and the manic states is, for the patients, an ineffable experience. It is absurd and intolerable; it clutters the whole area of thought and every piece of oneself. It is the inexorable passage for thinking, acting and feeling. Dehumanizing in that it prevents one from reaching what is essential in the human condition, suffering reminds patients that they cannot completely control their biological nature, perhaps because suffering confronts them with their own limits. Always undesirable, it can in some cases lead them, once the episode is resolved, to redefine their priorities by integrating their own fragility. Suffering is paradoxical because it is senseless and at the same time prone to make one think, but also because its overflowing presence is often followed by oblivion as soon as the patient heals. It nevertheless remains, for bipolar subjects who have experienced it, a terrorizing possibility that they wish to avoid at all costs. This is why, outside of an episode, many well-stabilised patients bear something like an invisible wound as a discreet and permanent apprehension, like a flaw in their unconcern.

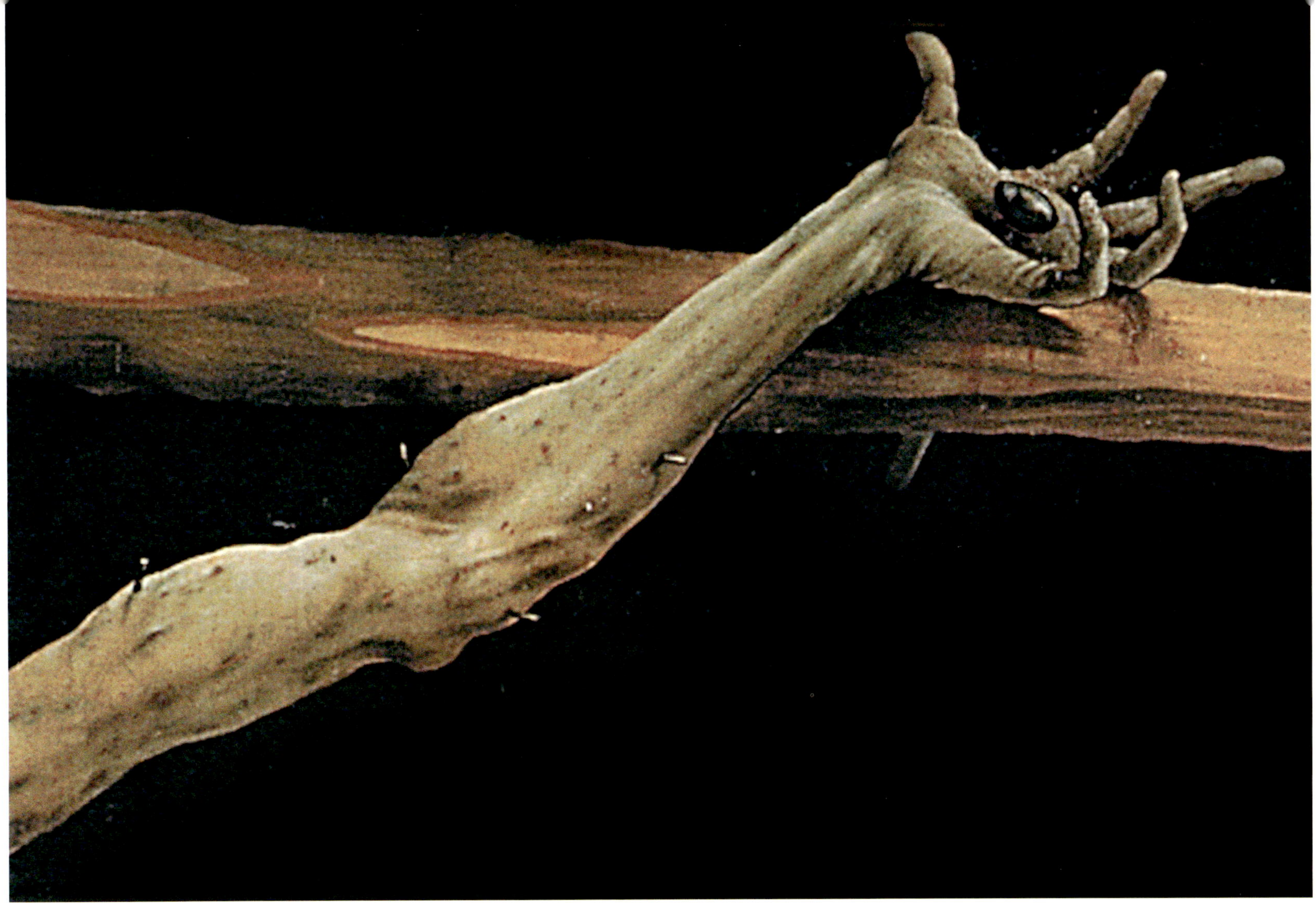

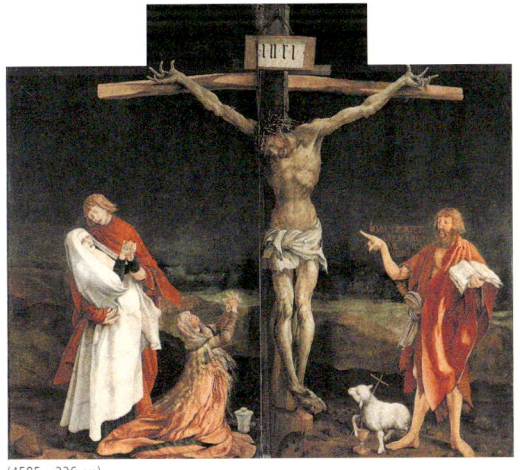

(4585 x 336 cm)

It is to the French writer Huysmans that we owe the rediscovery of **Matthias Grünewald** (circa 1475-1528), whose masterpiece, the Issenheim Altarpiece, can be seen today in Colmar, France, at the Unterlinden Museum. The altarpiece comprises five parts in all, four of which are painted on both sides, articulated around a wooden statuary, attributed to Nicolas Hagenau, representing the figures of three saints: Antonius, Augustinus and Hieronymus.

A contemporary of Dürer, Cranach the Elder and Holbein, Grünewald focused his creation on religious themes, to which he gave an amazingly expressionist interpretation, in contrast with the Medieval practices of the time.

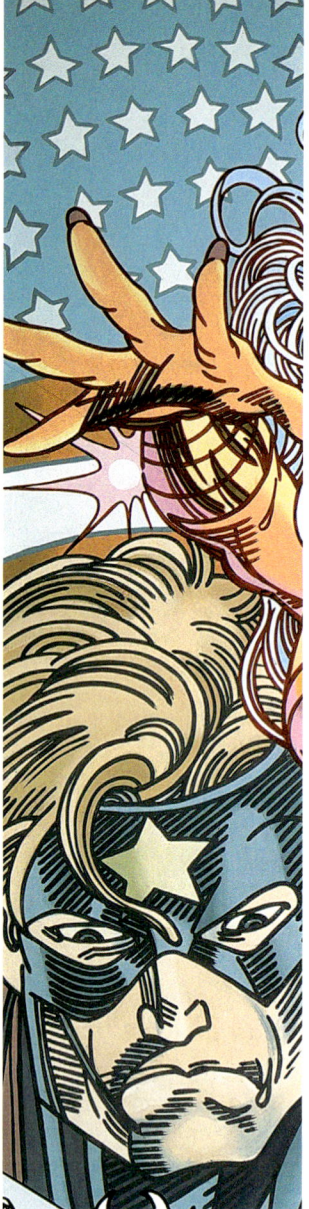

A hand soars from the canvas amidst triumphant forms. The woman these forms depict is a sex symbol, the archetype of a body bound to the stereotyped codes of seduction. Behind the woman's determined left fist stands her motionless pale-coloured mirror image, lost in her thoughts, with the American flag in the background. The character on the left, although of similar drawing technique, gives an insight into what is going on underneath it all. Tight-lipped and looking sombre, he is contemplating the disaster: the dislocated, tortured bodies of the victims of Guernica, Picasso's masterpiece, reproduced here by the artist in the predella. On the one hand, arrogant and colourful assurance; on the other, greyness, absurdity and death.

This painting juxtaposes opposite dimensions pushed to the extreme and makes them coexist in a subtle graphic and symbolic interlocking. The contrast is sharp between the triumphant assurance and the feeling of omnipotence by which the manic patient is driven and the doubt, the disorganisation and the despair by which the melancholic patient is overcome. Nevertheless, their joint presence in the same painting shows that these opposites are part of the same, single entity: bipolar disorder. Whatever the state, manic or depressive, a common feature of the disorder is its expression in excess and violence, breaking off from the surrounding world. This explains why, even outside of mixed states where symptoms of mania and depression are associated, we can sometimes discern pathos in the mania and excess in the melancholy.

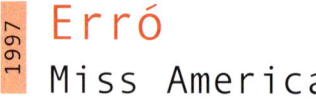

1997 **Erró**
Miss America

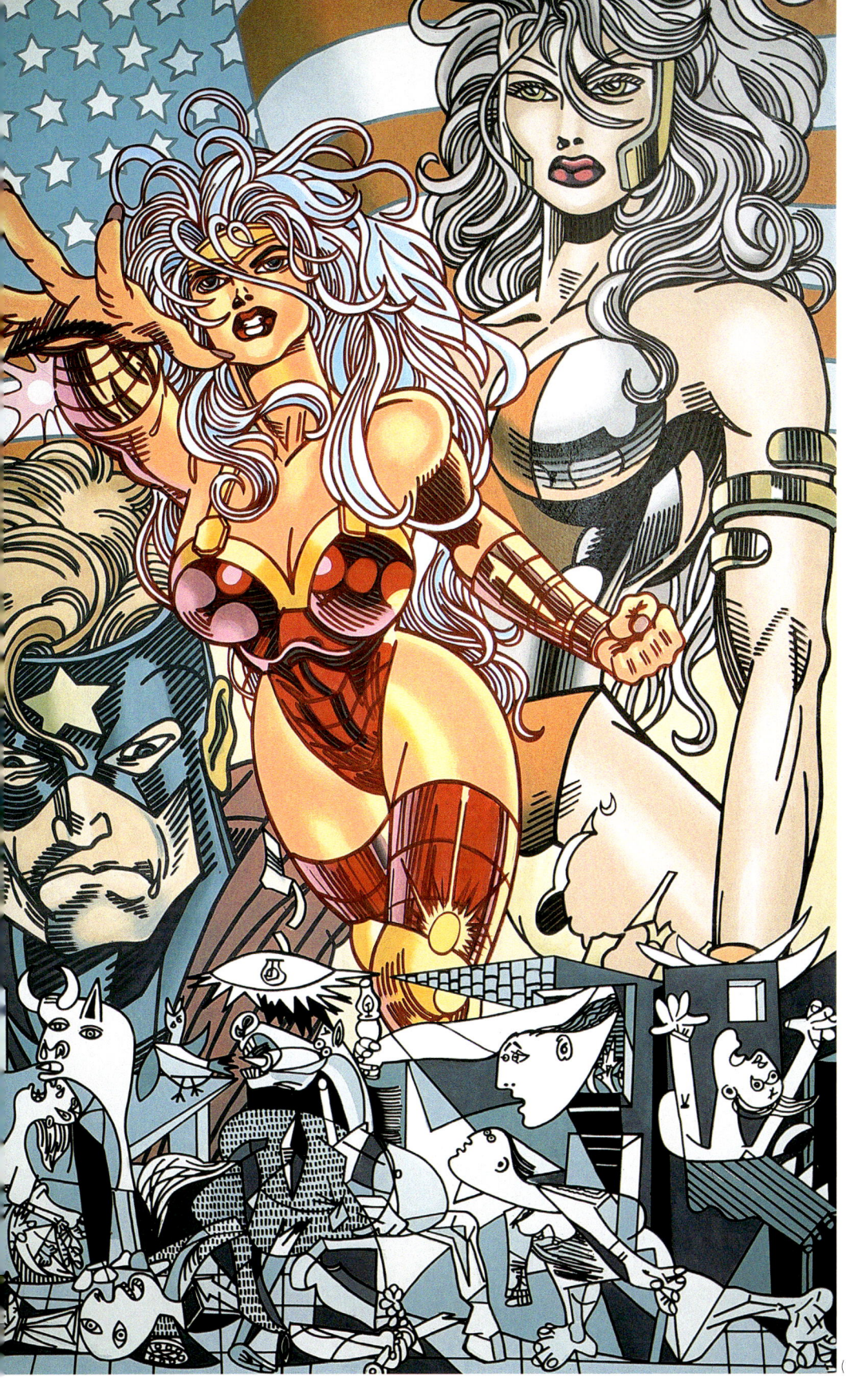

*The Icelandic artist **Erró**, whose real name is Gudmundur Gudmundsson, born in Olafsvik in 1932, began his career as mosaicist. His paintings, frequently associating strip-cartoon and science-fiction styles, are pictorial and political manifestos. "Painting is the laboratory of the possible," he has stated. Today, he spends his time between Paris, Thailand and Spain.*

(195 x 130 cm)

Bipolar Disorder: A Single Illness with Many Faces

A person affected by bipolar disorder can present, at intervals of several months (or years), episodes that are apparently completely different from each other. A first manifestation of the disorder can for instance appear in a person's late teens in the form of a seemingly isolated suicide attempt by an adolescent with persistent moroseness, in the context of a romantic break-up or scholastic failure. A few years later, the same person might present a state of excitement lasting for a few weeks, featuring extreme optimism, inconsiderate spending, insomnia and a sudden change in lifestyle. This radical change, although it may have entailed a sick leave or a romantic break-up and had manifest financial repercussions, may not only have been attributed to an outside cause, it may have also been deemed relatively unimportant because it quickly developed in a positive direction. Later – still with the same person – recurring depression might develop and require medicinal treatment. Another symptom such as anxiety might also arise over the years, and often precede depressive states. The diversity of the symptoms presented by the patient is such that it seems impossible – when studying the patient's case alone – to consider that these different episodes are the expression of a single illness. Any combination of symptoms can be seen in patients with bipolar disorder. For such patients taken singly, there is apparently nothing in common between those who have systematic relapses in the manic mode and those who have presented the symptoms of a manic state only once whereas all their other episodes are depressive. This explains why the disorder was so late in being identified (in the mid-nineteenth century), even though manic and depressive states had been described since the Antiquity.

Indeed, Hippocrates (circa 460-370 BC) had already delineated a mood state that he called melancholia ("black bile" in Greek), constituted of sadness and fear at the same time, the cognitive affliction of a state that later appeared to Claudius Galenus (AD 131-201), who had indicated at the time that melancholia was "*a kind of dotage without a fever, having for his ordinary companions, fear and sadness*" which damages thinking and provokes an aversion for what is most dear. Mania, for its part, was first considered in the Antiquity as a symptom (of the same type as fever) that could occur in different psychological disorders (including melancholia). It was then progressively individualised as a full-fledged disorder. Aretaeus of Cappadocia (AD 80-138) (3) observing the diversity of manic symptoms, wrote: "*There are infinite forms of mania,*" immediately adding: "*but the disease is one.*" He also mentioned the manic behaviour induced by psychotropic substances, in particular by wine, which in drunkenness could also inflame and make one delusional; the same, he said, was true of substances such as mandrake and henbane, but their effects were not called mania. He explained that in these cases, the effects came about suddenly and that return to composure was quick, whereas in mania they were firmly maintained.

In addition, he underscored the seasonal character of the mood disorder by describing the existence of patients appearing to be well and for whom their illness was reactivated in the spring. Long before Galenus, he mentioned the possible influence of the psychological disposition at work, between the episodes, in the type of mood disorder by which the patient might be affected. According to him, a certain type of temperament (the usual and stable psychological features of a given individual) was more likely to be connected with an evolution towards mania, whereas another would be more likely to move towards melancholy. Thus, certain persons, who were quick-tempered, prompt to excitement, who liked action, were easy to get along with, happy and enjoyed playing would be more inclined to be affected by a manic episode during this season. On the other hand, those who were nonchalant, sad, slow to learn but capable of enduring effort, he said, are more likely to fall into melancholy. Aretaeus described the behaviour and thinking disorders of manic patients as well as the repercussions of the state on public life: "*If mania is associated with joy, the patient may laugh, play, dance night and day, and go the market crowned as if victor in some contest of skill.*"

Two excerpts also show that Aretaeus of Cappadocia, like Alexander of Tralles later (in the sixth century), considered that there was a link between these two mood states. In the first, in which he describes the evolution of the symptoms of a manic patient, he mentions, among the many possible forms of evolution, one in which the mania evolves towards depression. Manic patients, he says, will then flee company for solitude, wish to be left to themselves and become listless, calm and sad. In a second passage, he indicates that melancholic patients, especially those in whom this disposition is confirmed, easily become manic, and that when the mania stops, the melancholy starts again; so that there is a to-and-fro from one to the other depending on the period (15).

It was not before the nineteenth century that two French authors, Jean Pierre Falret in 1854 (7, 16) who described "*la folie circulaire*" ("circular insanity") and, the same year, Jules Baillarger (4), who spoke of "*la folie à double forme*" ("dual-form insanity"), would describe the contours of the illness as we consider it today. According to Falret, it is characterized by the successive and regular evolution of the manic state, the melancholic state and a more-or-less prolonged lucid interval. (7). In the early twentieth century in Germany, Emil Kraepelin (10,11) would describe bipolar disorder under the name of Manic-depressive Psychosis in the eighth edition of his famous *Textbook of Psychiatry*. In particular, he isolated severe forms of depression that might feature delusion, sometimes with hallucinations and complaints about the body (Cotard's syndrome). It is, however, his individualisation of mixed states that constitute his most original contribution. Finally, starting in the 1960s, and following the work among others of Karl Leonhard (12), Jules Angst (2), Carl Perris (14) and George Winokur (18), the illness was individualised with the criteria in use today under the name of Bipolar Illness or Disorder.

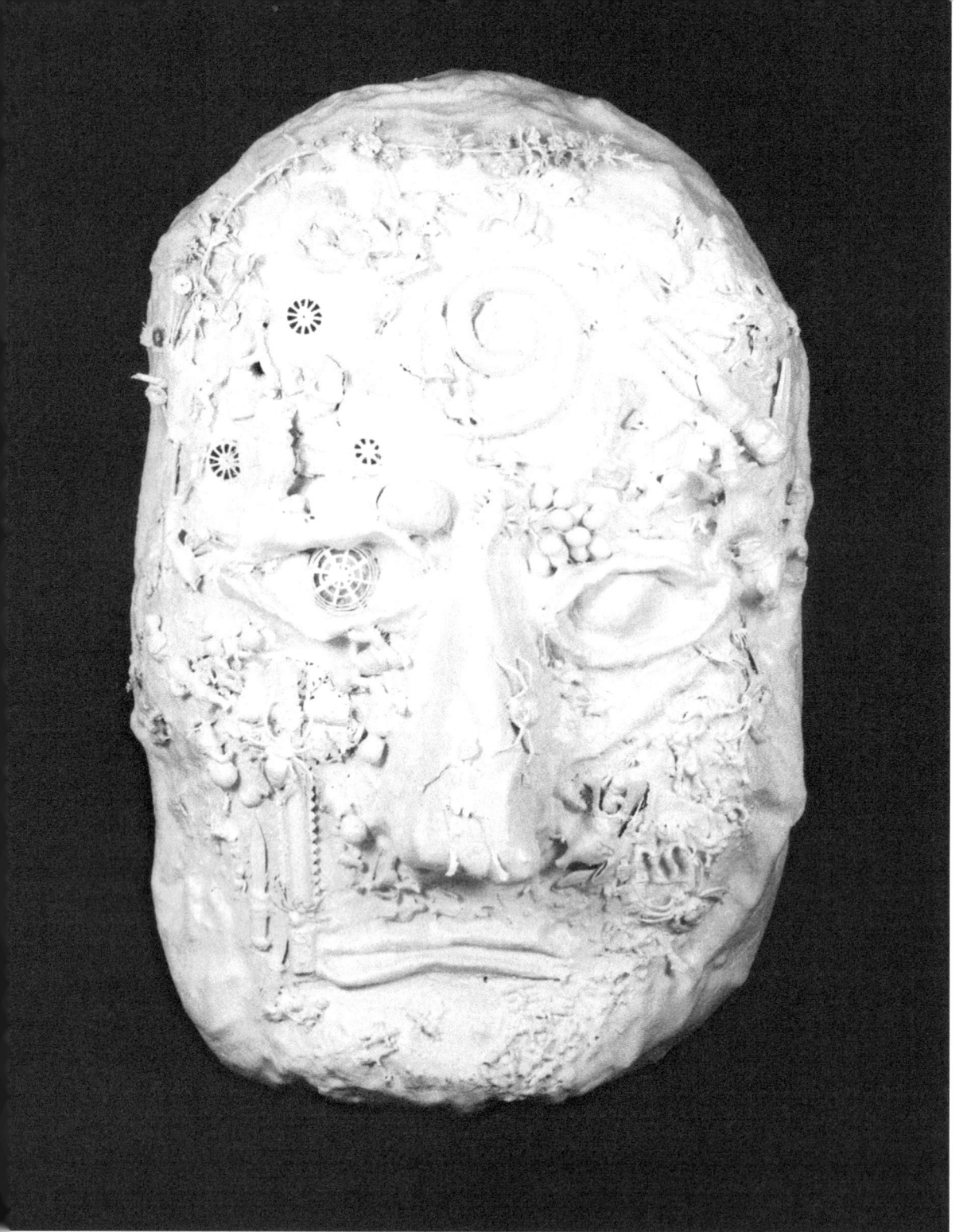

(125 x 80 x 37 cm)

*Born in France to a French father and an American mother, **Niki de Saint Phalle** (1930-2002) was a model before becoming the rousing artist that we know. An admirer of Gaudi and the Facteur Cheval, she decided early on to integrate objects into her work. Plastic figurines, little cars and other toys embrace the plaster in assemblages that are testimonies of the meeting of art and life. Inventor of the famous shooting of paint containers with a .22 calibre rifle, she excelled in the art of performance and proclaimed that a work of art is an "attack" and that she would "make the paint bleed". Her name remains connected to the Nanas, those large, round, colourful women in full bloom that she began to model in the sixties, and to that of Jean Tinguely, the Swiss artist who shared her life and her passion for creation.*

This head made of white plaster, lumpy with a multitude of reliefs, evokes an antique statue as much as a mortuary mask. The two forms of representation are culturally associated with a certain beauty, nobility and magnificence of the human condition. Looking for the harmony traditionally related to them, our gaze questions the details of the mask. And what do we make out? A disenchanted, tight-lipped mouth, a crushed nose inlayed with disturbing creatures: a skeleton, a beast, spider or crab, cancer in the middle of your face, death nipping at your nose. Reaching the eyes, our discomfiture grows: the right eye is staring at us, scrutinizing us, calling us with lucidity to testify to the pathetic terror of this face. The other eye is absent. There is no harmony here. This face reveals man in his least glorious reality, that of his finiteness and of his infinite solitude. The puffiness, an infiltrating disease, progressively alters the contours of the face. In the midst of the many inlays, a spiral on his front, a forgotten party streamer, is also a metaphor for the fleeing mind. The other objects — amputated swimmers, knives, miniature animals, fruits and plants, rose windows — appear like archaeological deposits brought to the surface by the effect of time. In the end, the face has no mask.

The melancholy state present in depressive periods is a phase of the disorder during which patients, in an apparent and frightening lucidity, solicit us at the same time that they are set in a too-late-anyway conviction. They call out when they know they are already lost, ruined, incurable. They spell out, often in infinite detail, the succession of the vicissitudes and dramas of their existence. Through this accumulation, they try to convince of the ineluctable nature of their progress towards death. Their body, perceived either as amputated of its organs (Cotard's syndrome) or as plagued by a malignant process (delusional hypochondria), is, in their eyes, proof of the active presence of death as much as of the impossibility of retaking their destiny into their own hands. In some cases, the punishment to which patients think they are submitted, like a castigation, is to survive their decomposition in complete lucidity without death's actually coming to abridge their suffering.

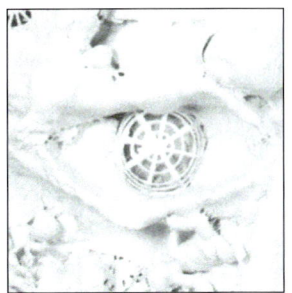

1964 **Niki de Saint-Phalle**
Gilles de Rais

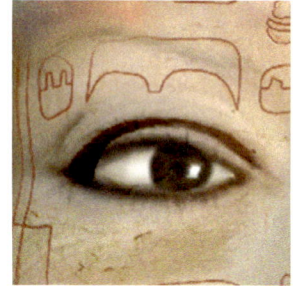

Orlan's regular-featured face, framed in a short bob reminiscent of a Soviet dancer's hairdo, is smiling. Her exaggerated makeup, recalling that of an American film star of the fifties, makes the apparent classicism of the photograph even stronger. The lines on her face are drawn with almost technological precision. They evoke the preliminary marks of an extremely ambitious plastic-surgery operation as much as they do the ritual drawings of a pre-Columbian mask or the enigmatic network of a computer chip. Two symmetrical bumps on her temples testify to the previous insertion of two of subcutaneous implants, deliberately introduced by the artist into her own face.

Orlan's face embodies modernity and the eternity of the body at the same time. The body here is an object of the world that can be changed at will, but also the manifestation of one's self given once and for all, a situation that is similar for every human body. Orlan thus transgresses and magnifies the cultural relationship to the body, which is both the material and the subject of her work, as well as instigator of the art work itself. The face thus staged and fixed in a photo, just like the face that she shows, live, in a video broadcast while she is undergoing plastic surgery, manifests the artist's determination to control time and the image. Nevertheless, the body changes that she can decide to make – or not – tells us that to know her, we should not trust this appearance. At any moment, a skilled lancet or some picture-touch-up software can show us a different image of her.

The patient's body fully participates in manic or depressive symptomatology just as much as emotion and thinking do. In the manic patient, the body in incessant movement, apparently insensitive to fatigue, displays its impatience to do even more, to enter into new adventures. It also participates in a desire to inform. While the easy motor functioning with ample gestures is indeed a reflection of the projects that the subject wishes to carry out, it also conveys non-verbal information. The body becomes an additional and polysemic channel through which manic patients attempt to communicate at the same time that they speak. In the abundance of ideas that are emerging, the body attempts to convey all that was not said for lack of time or of others' attention: the body too is logorrheic. In the depressed patient, the body testifies to the painful stopping of mental processes. Nonetheless, whereas words can cease when one believes one has no more to say, the body, which remains present, is always expressing something. Slowed-down, or even at a standstill as if struck with stupor, in melancholic states the body thus imposes itself on the ailing subject like a senseless hindrance. Either partially subtracted as in Cotard's syndrome or present but in pain as in hypochondria, the body of a depressed patient testifies, as much as the feeling of emptiness and pointlessness does, to the painful stopping of mental processes. The patient's body is like an object submitted to the unpredictable turns of the illness and cannot be discarded. Inconstant, in turn a driving force and an obstacle, an incarnation and a prison, a bipolar's body shows a multiplicity of representations of the subject. When is it itself? Always a little, but never completely. An impossible crossroads of a kind, the body is both the object and the subject of the patient's suffering.

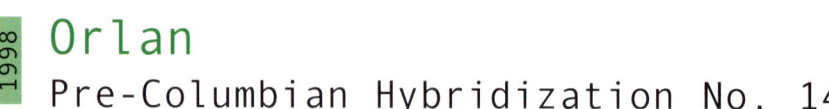

1998 Orlan
Pre-Columbian Hybridization No. 14

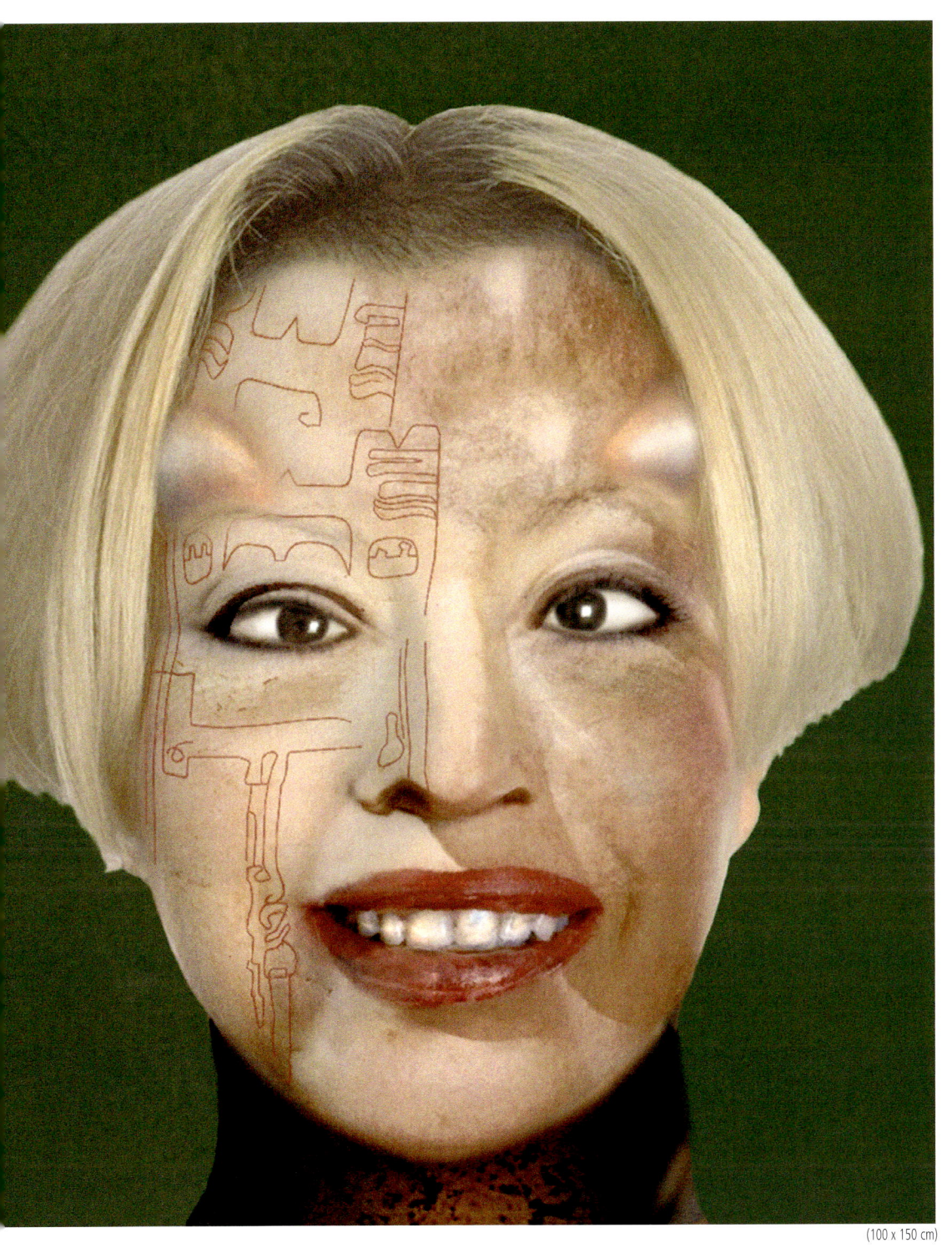

(100 x 150 cm)

*A proteiform and multidisciplinary plastic artist, **Orlan**, born in 1947, uses sculpture, photography, performance, video and multimedia as well as scientific technology (surgery and biogenetics) in the perpetual modelling and reshaping of her own body, producing a sort of real and virtual morphing to which she gives endless new expressions.*

Questioning our body's position in society, she transcends the woman's image and offers a redefinition of the Beautiful. The physical transformations are only the starting point of an approach that tends to endanger the very principle of identity. The first artist to use surgery as a medium, Orlan shows astonishing control, even in the most extreme of her actions.

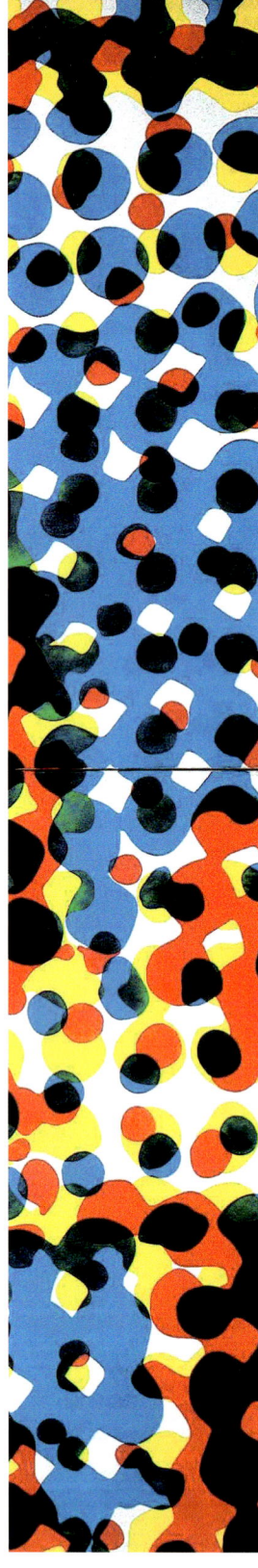

The points of colour covering the canvas, isolated primary colours, are blended or juxtaposed. They suggest the ultimate enlargement of a digital photo. The irregular contours of the colourful circles, sometimes connected, also call to mind red globules or cells in the process of division.

The extreme enlargement of the image, like that which makes the biological microscopic world visible, leads to the loss of perception of the whole object under study. Although represented in its most minute details, its presence is no longer perceptible. The – almost indiscreet – access to the intimate, the briefly perceived unsuspected immensity of the world, the suggestion of blood and reproduction, are striking. They generate a sensory and symbolic influx that makes viewers lose their references and plunges them into perplexity.

During manic states, hyper-vigilance to minute details leads the subject to perceive the world not as a whole, but as a mosaic of intense stimuli. Every stimulus is taken singly from the others and works as a whole; in addition, the subject grasps this totality as secreting some essential content. No concession, no relativity is therefore possible within this multitude of fragments of reality. The manic patient's world is thus constituted by an assemblage of percepts, all of them essential, with no priority to classify them by order of importance. The unity of the perceived situation and even the subject who experiences it can therefore not be grasped in its entirety. Every detail perceived thus takes on its own life and becomes a world in itself, autonomous from the whole that it belongs to. Attacked by a stream of sensory pieces of information that are partly detached from the context that engendered them, the manic patient perceives the objects and situations of the world as sensory abundance, often exulting but also disquieting because mixed into a world that has lost the unity and order of common reality.

Alain Jacquet
Portrait of a Woman, Jeannine
1965

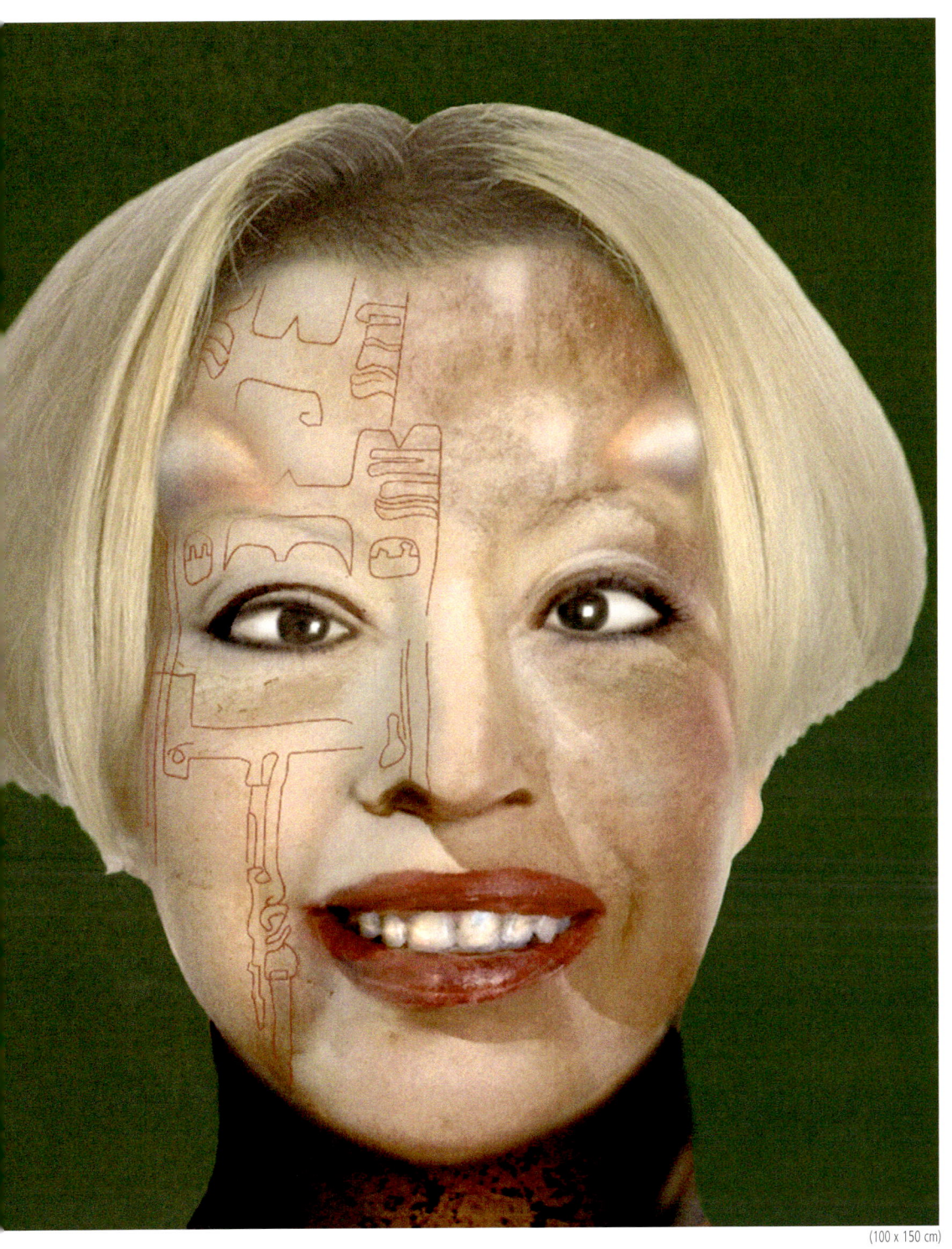

(100 x 150 cm)

*A proteiform and multidisciplinary plastic artist, **Orlan**, born in 1947, uses sculpture, photography, performance, video and multimedia as well as scientific technology (surgery and biogenetics) in the perpetual modelling and reshaping of her own body, producing a sort of real and virtual morphing to which she gives endless new expressions.*
Questioning our body's position in society, she transcends the woman's image and offers a redefinition of the Beautiful. The physical transformations are only the starting point of an approach that tends to endanger the very principle of identity. The first artist to use surgery as a medium, Orlan shows astonishing control, even in the most extreme of her actions.

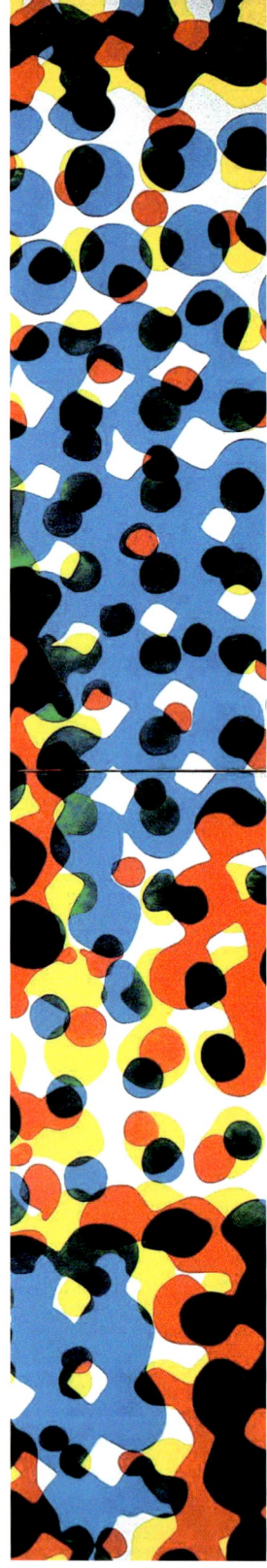

The points of colour covering the canvas, isolated primary colours, are blended or juxtaposed. They suggest the ultimate enlargement of a digital photo. The irregular contours of the colourful circles, sometimes connected, also call to mind red globules or cells in the process of division.

The extreme enlargement of the image, like that which makes the biological microscopic world visible, leads to the loss of perception of the whole object under study. Although represented in its most minute details, its presence is no longer perceptible. The – almost indiscreet – access to the intimate, the briefly perceived unsuspected immensity of the world, the suggestion of blood and reproduction, are striking. They generate a sensory and symbolic influx that makes viewers lose their references and plunges them into perplexity.

During manic states, hyper-vigilance to minute details leads the subject to perceive the world not as a whole, but as a mosaic of intense stimuli. Every stimulus is taken singly from the others and works as a whole; in addition, the subject grasps this totality as secreting some essential content. No concession, no relativity is therefore possible within this multitude of fragments of reality. The manic patient's world is thus constituted by an assemblage of percepts, all of them essential, with no priority to classify them by order of importance. The unity of the perceived situation and even the subject who experiences it can therefore not be grasped in its entirety. Every detail perceived thus takes on its own life and becomes a world in itself, autonomous from the whole that it belongs to. Attacked by a stream of sensory pieces of information that are partly detached from the context that engendered them, the manic patient perceives the objects and situations of the world as sensory abundance, often exulting but also disquieting because mixed into a world that has lost the unity and order of common reality.

Alain Jacquet
Portrait of a Woman, Jeannine
1965

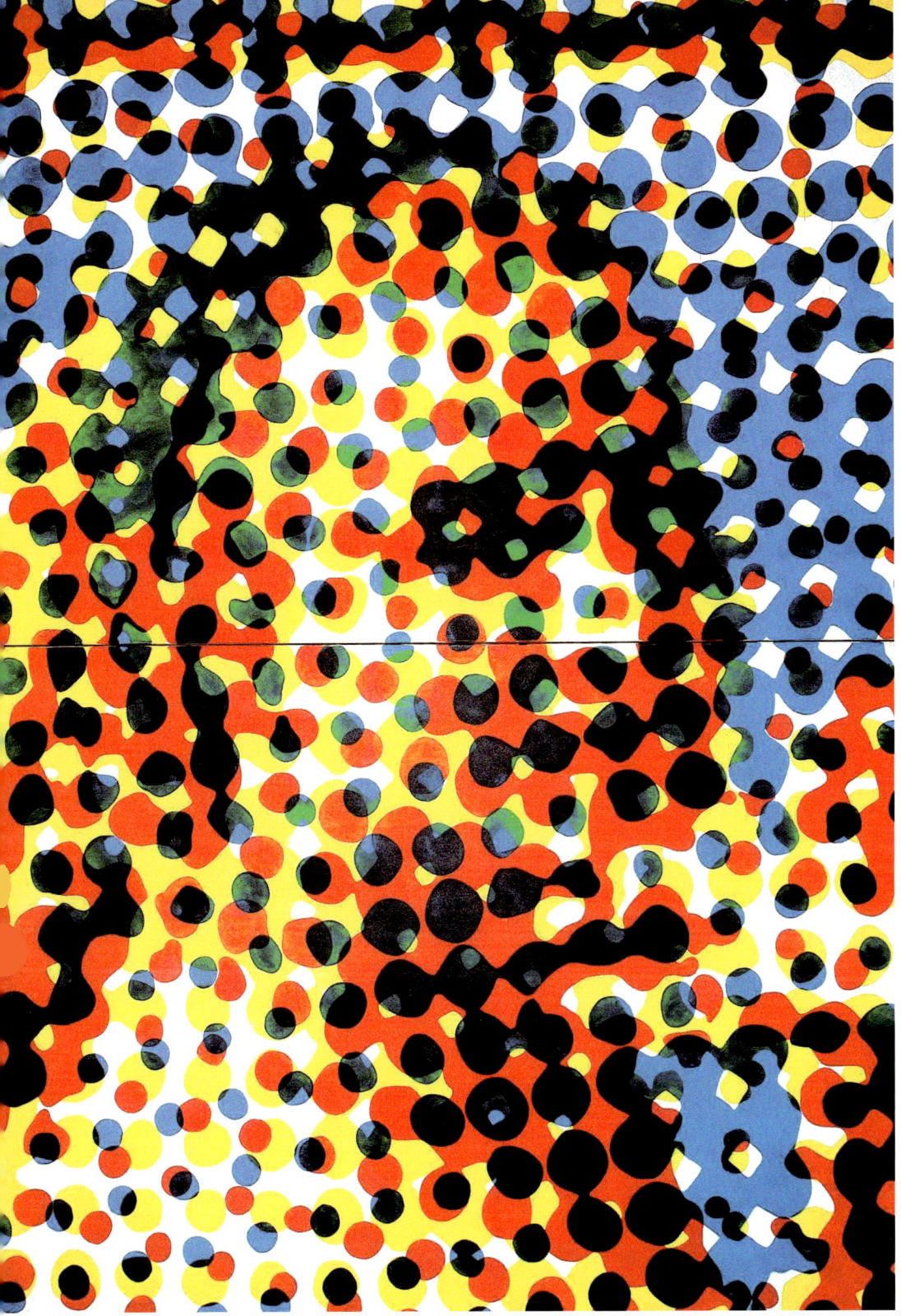

Born in Neuilly-sur-Seine in 1939, the French artist **Alain Jacquet** studied at the École des Beaux-arts in Paris. In 1964, with Mimmo Rotella, he created Mec Art, or screened photomechanical painting. All of his work being placed in the continuity of art history, it is not unlikely that through this technique, he was trying to resume the impressionists' small strokes of colour, or even with those of the pointillists. This is demonstrated for example by his re-interpretation of Manet's "Luncheon on the Grass". His peculiar way of dissecting images, of re-reading them, enhances the power of the context. The spot of colour is practically alone on the canvas, but it is linked to all the others through a screen, however infinitesimal. He reminds us that it derives all of its meaning exclusively from its relationship with the other spots of colour.

Alain Jacquet spends his time between Paris and New York.

(in two parts, 130 x 195 cm each)

– LOSS OF UNITY – HYPER-VIGILANCE TO DETAIL – DECONTEXTUALISATION – LOSS OF UNITY – HYPER-VIGILANCE TO

40

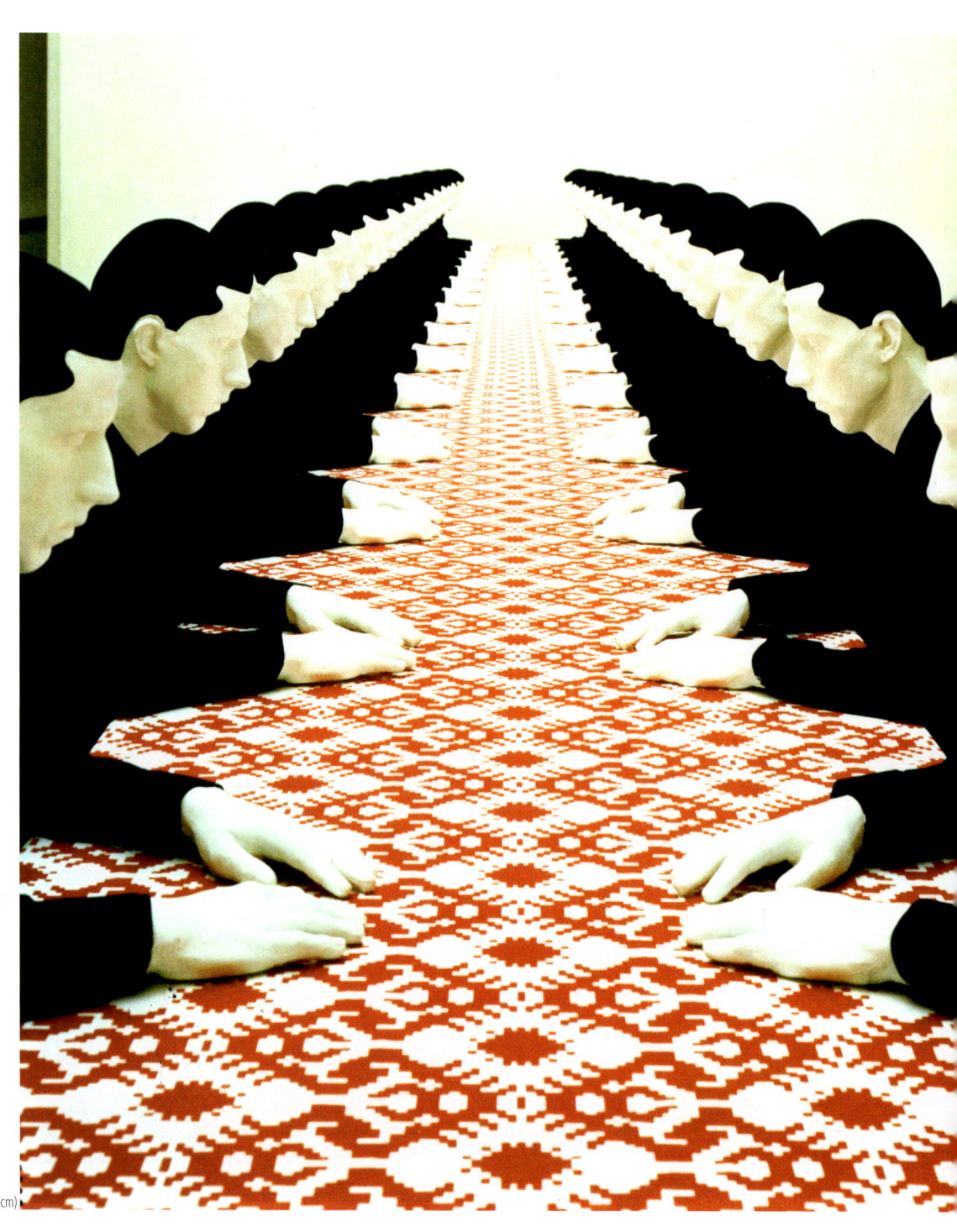

1988 Katharina Fritsch
Company at the Table

(141 x 1600.04 x 172.72/198.12 cm)

The thirty-two characters staged by Katharina Fritsch seem identical and lost in their thoughts. Motionless, their hands on the table, their back slightly hunched, looking downwards, they seem absorbed in themselves. The white of their flesh and the black of their hair and shirt conjure up a uniform and cleanliness as well as absence. In obvious contrast, the red-patterned tablecloth gives, for a moment, an illusion of fantasy. But we are soon won over by the likeness in the fractal repetition of geometric patterns and the mirror-positioned characters.

The expression on their faces and the position of their hands and bodies suggests that thinking is in progress. But the repetition and the fixedness of the poses leads us to imagine that even the thinking is made of repetitions. The thinking of one who is depressed is driven by mental processes made of pessimistic ideas, which, although they appear in succession according to an apparently linear logic, do not move forward because, having surreptitiously gone off track, they are caught in a loop. Although the mental activity of depressed patients is highly altered in terms as much of memory as of concentration, or more generally speaking of their ability to understand life, it is relentless and never leaves them alone. Their pessimistic preoccupations are not so much the result of the analysis of a thought process moving towards negative conclusions as of the emotional charge that the thinking contains. They believe they are thinking, but in fact they are feeling emotions. Everything happens as if their pessimistic ideas, which upset them and which they often consider as an "objective" reading of reality, constituted the material of logical reasoning, when they are only the repetition, related to different objects, of the same emotion: unhappiness.

So naturally, despite its constancy, a depressed person's "reasoning" does not work. Going nowhere, but pressed by a strong emotional charge, its unceasing repetition makes it possible to some extent to be under the impression of remaining active. The pre-established progress of closed thinking does not usually allow one who is depressed to be accessible to outside ideas, those of his familiar circles in particular. This repetition can be seen as a neurobiological anomaly and as a struggle against ideas of death as well. Isolated in their thoughts, impervious to outside solicitations, depressed patients remain hieratically alone in their non-transcendent world.

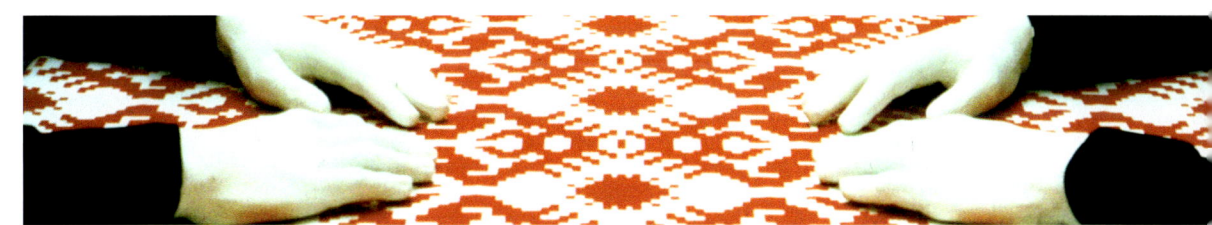

Katharina Fritsch *is German. She was born in 1956 and currently lives in Düsseldorf. Associating traditional sculpture and industrial production techniques, she is interested in the connection between reality and appearance, likes to plays on the tension between the familiar and the unusual and enjoys exploring the shadowy areas of the collective unconscious.*

The Bipolar's Palette

As for any other illness, bipolar disorder is rarely expressed in its pure form. Indeed, the sequence in which an abruptly developed manic state is followed by a severe depressive state – from which a patient totally recovers before being thrown again into the same manic-then-depressive cycle – is an exceptional occurrence.

In reality, a large number of clinical variants are possible. There are patients who never suffer from depression and who relapse only in the manic mode, whereas others, who have only had a single episode of an attenuated form of mania (hypomania) – sometimes having escaped observation – seem to be merely afflicted by chronic depression. Some patients will relapse very occasionally whereas others will suffer more than four episodes per year (rapid cycling). There are also patients in which one observes, especially in the manic forms, a mixture of signs of mania and signs of depression (mixed states). Seasons seem portentous to some (seasonal affective disorder) whereas for others a relapse seems utterly uncertain. For other patients, the development of a dependence (on alcohol in particular) is an equivalent of the mood disorder. Some bipolars also know that their behaviour can become completely extravagant during an episode and that it places them in contradiction with the values they stand for when they are well. For others, the delusions or hallucinations settle in as soon as they relapse. Among these latter, there is a small group of patients for whom recovery between the episodes is only partial (schizo-affective disorder).

Hypomania

Hypomania is an attenuated form of mania. Instead of the extravagant or dishevelled clothing and the continuous movement and agitation of the manic patient, one observes in the hypomanic patient a non-conformist appearance and great ease in contacts with others with an above-average energy. The acceleration of thoughts in manic patients (tachypsychia) in which ideas pour in, unstable and expressed through unceasing wordplay, is replaced in the hypomanic patient by an impression of extreme ease in thinking and an abundance of ingenious ideas, like a momentary excess of creativeness. The mood exaltation with excessive self-confidence, unrealistic or megalomanic projects of the manic patient is replaced in the hypomanic patient by optimism and the pleasure of living. The sometimes total insomnia of the manic patient is substituted in the hypomanic patient by an impression of quick, restoring sleep.

In the child and the teenager, hypomania can be expressed by accesses of anger, a sudden emotional upheaval, hyperactivity, attention disorders, discipline problems at school or risk behaviour.

Rapid Cycling

Certain bipolar patients are afflicted by a very rapid alternation of thymic episodes: this is called rapid cycling. In some cases, it is so rapid that there are practically no free intervals between the episodes. Three different types of this form are differentiated: rapid cycling ($\geq$ 4/year), ultra-rapid cycling ($\geq$ 4/month) and ultradian cycling (distinct episodes within a 24-hour period). These forms are to be distinguished from cyclothymia, a state where the mood fluctuates but never actually reaches either mania or depression. Nonetheless, rapid cycling should not be reduced to a simple acceleration of recurrences (like music with a faster beat); it should rather suggest mood instability, as if the passage from one thymic state to another had been made easier. Bipolar patients with rapid cycling do not usually remain in this state for long. Many risk factors for moving into a rapid-cycling mode have been proposed. Some authors suggest that having a cyclothymic temperament before the beginning of the disorder favours the advent of rapid cycling. Others indicate that this characteristic is more frequent in women; indeed, most studies show that 70 to 92% of rapid-cycling patients are women. There is also more frequent substance abuse in rapid-cycling bipolar patients. Anti-depressants taken alone, i.e., without the prescription of an associated mood stabiliser (such as lithium) could also favour the advent of rapid cycling.

```
COMME L'ON
S'AMUSE
        BI
        EN

    les
    heures
```

Two objects are formed by the words placed on the white page: a tie and a fob watch. Incongruous materials for two customary objects. The text is reminiscent of the automatic writing so dear to the Surrealists. Words of scholarly resonance are mixed into words used in the language of everyday life. The winder of the watch, a Cyclops or a smile, might be the key to this rebus: *on s'amuse*, we're having fun. The words are pearls, dropped and threaded to the liking of the poet's pranks. Those paradigms of social convention, time and a tie, are mocked in a subtly caustic manner, because the tool for this derision is conventional par excellence: words. This invitation to shake off the yoke of social constraint is summed up entirely in the first text: "*LA CRAVATE DOULOUREUSE QUE TU PORTES ET QUI T'ORNE Ô CIVILISÉ ÔTE-LA SI TU VEUX BIEN RESPIRER*": THE PAINFUL TIE THAT YOU WEAR AND DECORATES YOU OH CIVILISED ONE TAKE IT OFF IF YOU WISH TO BREATHE WELL. The message of the watch text, which can be read in one direction or the other, is not the result of a significant succession of logically connected words, it emerges from the incongruity of their juxtaposition.

Such use of words, where they are not exclusively at the service of sentences but take on a life of their own through their verve, their metaphor or their extravagance is what constitutes manic discourse. Word play, unexpected associations and a caustic approach to conventions all add up to an apparently constructed, both immediate and hermetic language. There is also in the manic patient a true playing with language: everything is an excuse for mockery. A situation that is being experienced, for example, is abundantly and vividly described in real time: it is examined from its most derisive angle, pointing to the comic detail or highlighting what convention usually expects not to be said. In the manic patient, words often follow one another in such a way that one word leads to another not in terms of the general meaning of the sentence but using, for a given word, another of its possible meanings. It is also through assonance or metaphor that the transition from one word to another can take place. Not only changeable and sparkling, a manic patient's language sometimes surprises by its unexpected digressions and fascinates in the brio of its semantic associations. This fireworks of language is considered by patients as the testimony of sharpness, intelligence, and an absolute power of seduction; thus, it participates in their impression of omnipotence. Nonetheless, manic patients, whose language expresses a mayhem of hurried ideas, all of them bearing essence but instantly swept away, stage in their discourse a fundamentally unstable character. Very often, when we are listening to them, we wonder: "Who is speaking, by the way?"

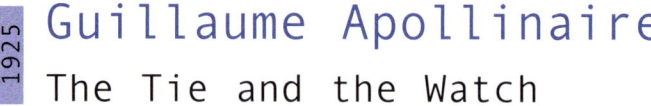

Guillaume Apollinaire
1925
The Tie and the Watch

La cravate et la montre

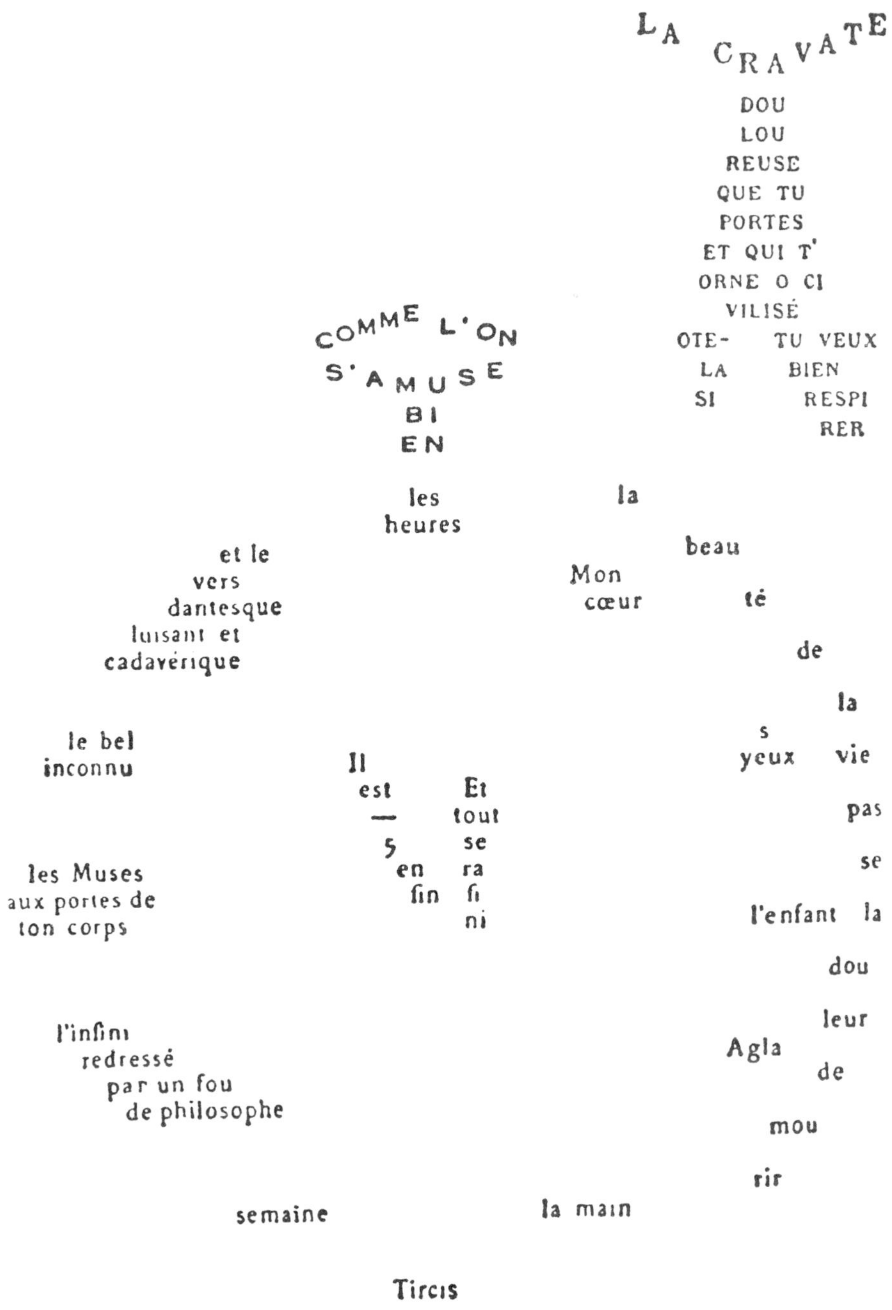

```
              LA
            CRAVATE
             DOU
             LOU
             REUSE
             QUE TU
             PORTES
             ET QUI T'
             ORNE O CI
             VILISÉ
          OTE-    TU VEUX
           LA      BIEN
  COMME L'ON
  S'AMUSE    SI      RESPI
     BIEN             RER
      EN
```

les heures

la

beau

Mon cœur

té

et le
vers
dantesque
luisant et
cadavérique

de

la

s
yeux   vie

le bel
inconnu

Il
est   Et
—   tout
5   se
  en ra
  fin fi
       ni

pas

se

l'enfant la

les Muses
aux portes de
ton corps

dou

leur

Agla   de

l'infini
  redressé
    par un fou
      de philosophe

mou

rir

semaine   la main

Tircis

*It was in 1918 that the poet and art critic **Guillaume Apollinaire** created the word "calligram" to name those lyrical ideograms in which drawings and poems keep complex, subtle and plural relations. The invention of these "art games" is most certainly not foreign to Apollinaire's friendship with the greatest painters of his time: Derain, Picasso, Sonia and Robert Delaunay, to mention just a few. They also reflect the poet's taste for typography – he did his own printing with a hand press.*

Whether Sophie Calle is taking photographs of people who were born blind and then places, next to their faces – which the subjects themselves have never seen – texts in which they tell how they imagine beauty, whether she is showing us the places visited by an anonymous person that she has secretly followed in Venice or whether she is recording the rooms in luxury hotels where she has got herself hired as a chamber woman, her productions (photos and often texts) always show absence and presence at the same time. An archaeologist of contemporary times, she seizes, indiscreetly as much as ingenuously, a reality where there is no one, but that still bears the traces of the person who has gone. Everything happens as if knowledge of others could be understood in a more "objective" – although limited – way after they have left. As if their actual presence, inasmuch as it clutters our subjectivity, made them less visible in their truth. Sophie Calle's work thus solicits us in a reconstruction process, a process for the representation of others on the basis of the recent remains of their presence in reality. A classic variation of the image or mirror theme, her work is paradoxically accomplished through the representation of absence. "The Tie" goes one step further in this approach, as this is no longer the photograph of a hotel room after its occupant has gone out; it is the creation from scratch of a hotel room abandoned by a client who has never existed. The verisimilitude of the scene in which the clothes are plausibly disposed by what we imagine to be a well-groomed man who has stayed at a luxury hotel, incite us to imagine him with the help of social archetypes and our own fantasies. Might he not just be delighting in carnal pleasures at the moment when the photo is being taken? The very real absence of an image of this phantom guest allows our imagination to grasp him and give him a life without having to adapt to the reality of his presence. There is nevertheless a nagging doubt: suppose we are mistaken?

Persons suffering from bipolar disorder often have trouble remembering their episodes once they are over. It is as if despite its intensity, the mental state expressed during the manic or depressive periods was of a different nature than the one they are in between the episodes. The difficulty to remember the symptoms, a form of absence from oneself within oneself, can be understood as a memory disorder and as an impasse in meaning as well. How, indeed, can we attribute an inner coherence to these manifestations fragmented by mania or shattered by depression? How, too, can we integrate them into the continuous thread of our life? Yet reconstituting these periods turns out to be indispensable, as much because of the need to maintain unity of self in the course of time as because the effectiveness of prophylactic treatment can only be conceived if the patient has integrated the succession of episodes as being part of the same, single disorder. A psychological reconstruction process proves therefore to be necessary between the episodes. On the one hand, it allows the patient to own the information on the disorder brought to light in a psycho-educational framework. On the other hand, it establishes during psychotherapy a representation of the "forgotten" past, which mixes elements of its reality with an imaginary reconstruction that thus becomes a signifying whole. Thus, like the viewer of Sophie Calle's work who attempts to solve the absence enigma, the bipolar patient reconstitutes the missing parts of the pathological periods. Here again, and like the texts of the blind solicited by Sophie Calle to speak of beauty and placed next to the photo of their face, the creation-remembering work comes to pass through words, the recounting of a self that has vanished and has become present once again.

Sophie Calle
1996 The Tie

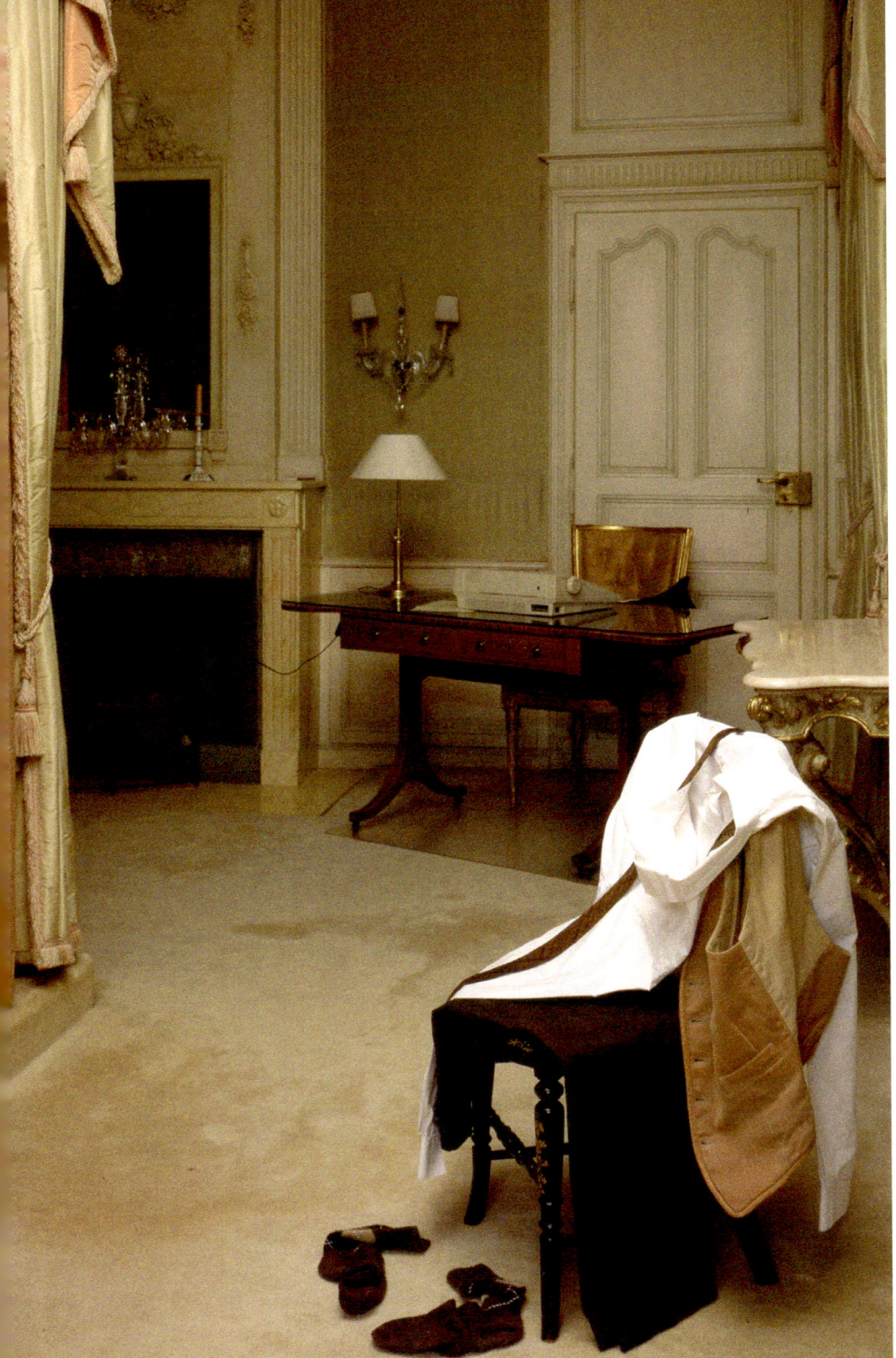

"The Tie

I saw him for the first time in December 1985, at a lecture he was giving. I found him attractive but one thing bothered me: he was wearing an ugly tie. The next day I anonymously sent him a thin brown tie. Later, I saw him in a restaurant; he was wearing it. Unfortunately, it clashed with his shirt. It was then I decided to take on the task of dressing him from head to toe: I would send him one article of clothing every year at Christmas. In 1986, he received a pair of silk grey socks; in 1987, a black alpaca sweater; in 1988, a white shirt; in 1989, a pair of gold-plated cufflinks; in 1990, a pair of boxer shorts with a Christmas tree pattern; nothing in 1991; and in 1992, a pair of grey trousers. Someday, when he is fully dressed by me, I would like to be introduced to him."

Sophie Calle *seeks reality in narration, which may be more tangible than our own life, through which we travel in absence. Sophie Calle, or the art of "telling about herself" and telling about others. It was during a love journey in the United States that her artistic career began, although she has declared to have been defined as an 'artist' by Bertrand Lamarche-Vadel, curator for the Paris Biennial of 1979. In the United Sates, in Venice, then in France, Sophie Calle found a thousand and one ways of narrating her life, "her stories" and finally those of others. Inviting friends and strangers, she photographed them while they were sleeping in her bed; she followed passers-by and snatched photos of them in a true investigation of anonymous intimacy.*

In the eighties, she could be seen strip-teasing in Pigalle but she was also a chamber woman in a hotel, the better to scrutinise and photograph the clients' personal belongings. Playing on the reality-fiction ambiguousness, Sophie Calle displays her life between performances and novels and ends up with a narrative-art approach in which fetishism, representation and voyeurism are mingled.

48

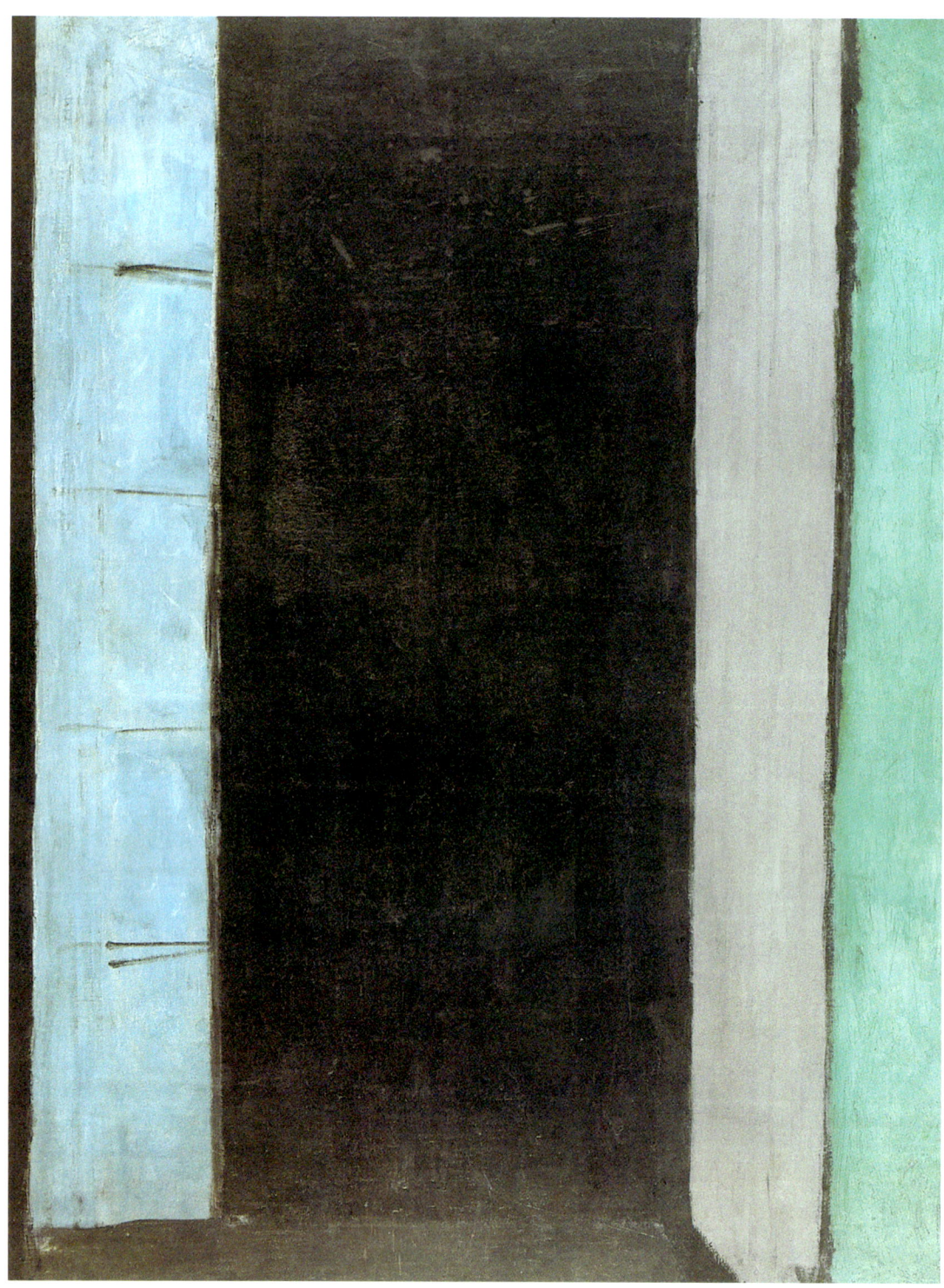

Henri Matisse
French Window in Collioure
1914

(1,165 x 89 cm)

49

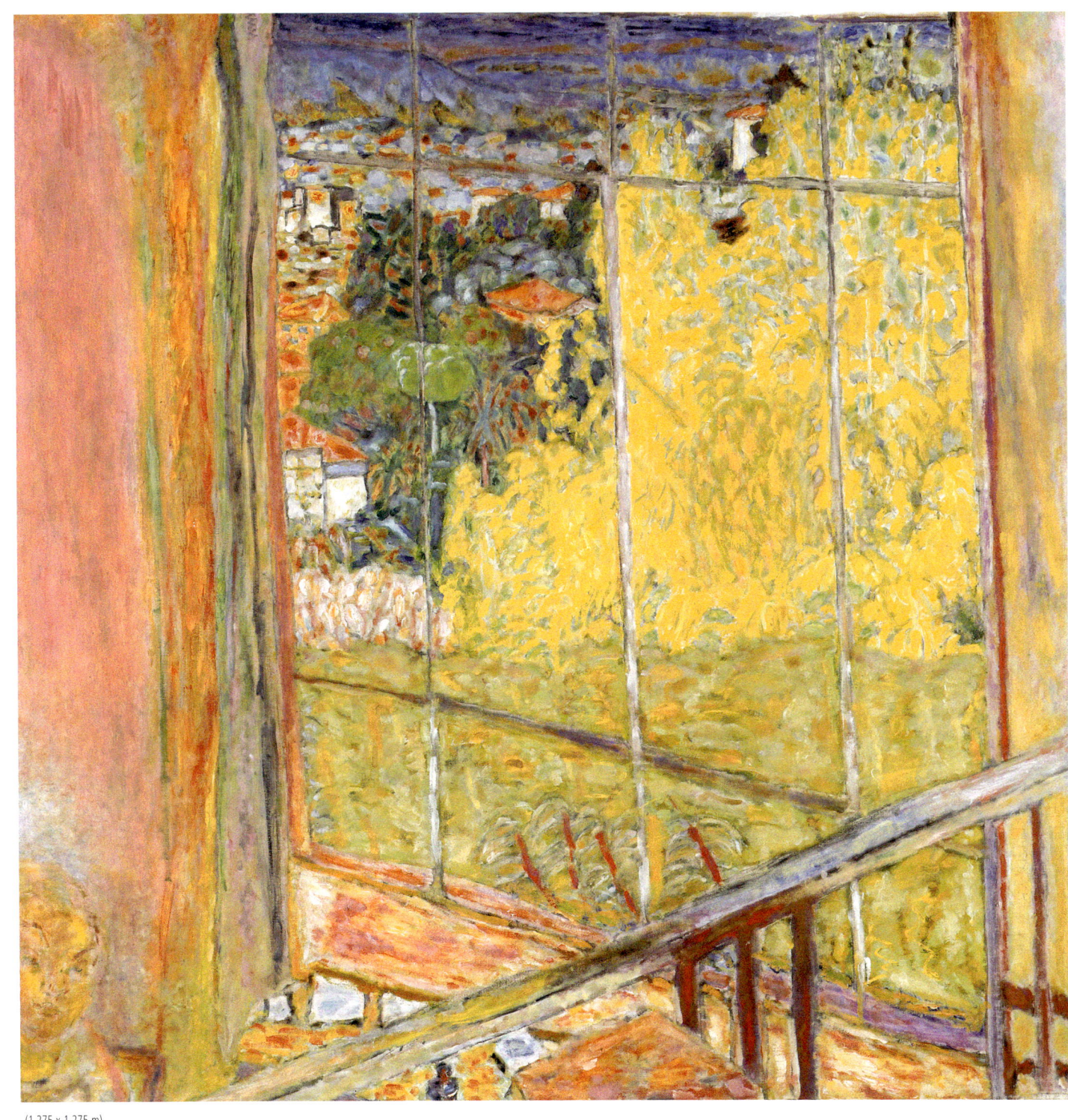

Pierre Bonnard
Studio with Mimosa
1939-1946

(1.275 x 1.275 m)

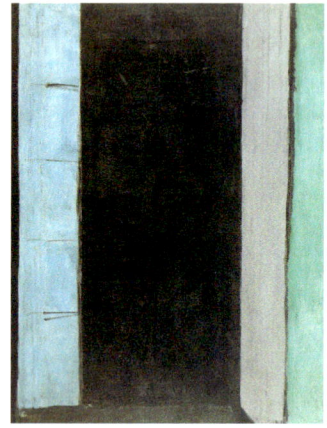

Henri Matisse
1914
French Window in Collioure

The rectangular canvas features three vertical strips in light hues framing a dark central area. An odd French window, indeed! The dark recess under the left-hand strip invites us to penetrate further but the darkness is an immediate obstacle. The streaks on the right in soft colours, reminiscent of fluid curtains, establish the moving limits of the viewer's place. Naturally attracted, one would like to go farther. But the dull opacity disillusions one's expectation: nothing, there is no beyond. The curtains freeze and seem to become mineral columns or bars on the window… one cannot go any farther.

Pierre Bonnard
1939-46
Studio with Mimosa

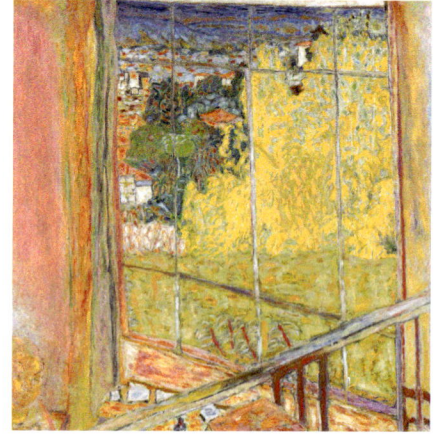

The huge square canvas is splashed with yellow. It imposes itself like an all-encompassing blanket and takes possession of the landscape. Omnipresent, almost intoxicating, it penetrates the painter's studio. The window and the railing are powerless to keep out the sensory tide that is setting a fire inside. In the distance, the cold colours suggest that this blinding effusion is occurring in the middle of winter. Inside – we can feel it – the temperature is mild. The glass partition of the studio protects from the cold and from the night, which is falling. On the left, a woman, a red silhouette on a red background, is barely visible, as if blended into the setting. And yet her presence is radiant. Just as the painter's, whom we cannot see but whose sensitivity we perceive all over.

These two highly contrasted paintings question a common and fundamental dimension of the bipolar patient: his trouble in establishing the proper boundary. The boundary that defines the inside and the outside, self and others. With Matisse, the apparently open window opens onto nothingness and sends you back to the world's immobility and to infinite solitude. With Bonnard, the outside comes inside, warms you up and suggests the sensitive presence of others. But you don't want to go outside because it's cold out. In both perspectives, circulation between the inside and the outside, self and others, is one-way. The powerlessness to be part of the world or, on the contrary, the impression of being invaded by it illustrates the patient's boundary disorder, present as much in his depressive as in his manic phases. Depressed patients who experience their life as cut off from the world and as isolated in the heart of their ontological solitude feel nevertheless so fragile that the surrounding world seems to them intrusive and dangerous. They say they prefer to protect themselves from it whereas they suffer from not being able to be part of it. As with Matisse, they dream of being able to go out the window that they see ajar. But as soon as they approach it, they are seized by the harshness of the life outside and by the opacity of its intelligibility. Manic patients, on the other hand, feel that all that surrounds them is familiar and thus they authorise themselves to intrude in the world of others. They interfere with inappropriate comments or actions, which they judge to be legitimate because of their all-encompassing certainty of the superiority of their understanding. Not only inopportune because they often do not grasp what has commanded others' actions, but also disagreeable because they get in the way of others' autonomy, manic patients are tiresome and irritating. This leads them to being rejected into the coldness of a landscape without others. To the patient's active exclusion is added that which comes from himself: judging his familiar circles to be too slow and too conservative, he decides to make do without them. Thus, though they see themselves in the heart of the world, manic patients are doubly excluded from it, by themselves and by others. To establish the right relational distance is therefore a difficult task as much for the depressed as for the manic patient.

Before settling in the south of France and becoming the painter of a luminous and colour-saturated daily life, **Pierre Bonnard** *(1867-1947) was one of the leading figures of the Nabis. The Nabis (Hebrew for "prophets") were a group of a dozen young painters in the 1890s who were keen on inventing a new form of painting – decorative and drawing largely from Japanese art.*

For **Henri Matisse** *(1869-1954), the painter of colour and elegantly pleasing harmonious shapes, this is an unusual painting. After having participated in the great Fauve adventure alongside Derain, Manguin, Marquet and Vlaminck, amongst others, Matisse undertook a sensitive and deliberately decorative pictographic quest, which he inventively pursued in the large paper cut-outs that he created at the end of his life. "I feel through colour," he would say.*

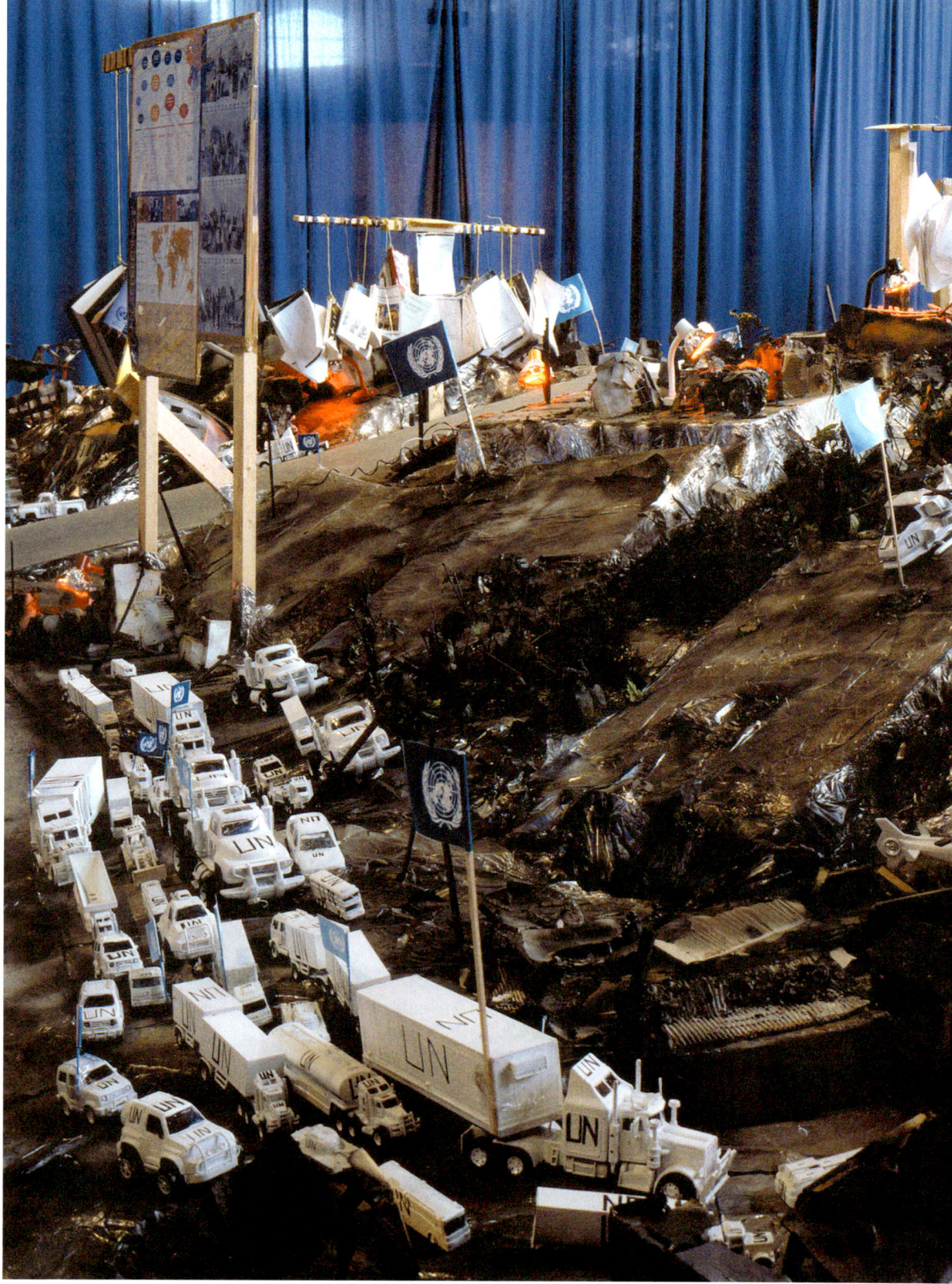

*Born in 1957, the Swiss artist **Thomas Hirschhorn** declares that his work is "socially committed". "My choice was to refuse to make political art," he says, "I make art politically." He finds our consumption society to be too full of objects, words and images that change or ineluctably induce a loss of meaning, of symbol. He therefore focuses on emptiness, the debris of consumerism and disappearance.*

Linking up the innumerable elements constituting his installations with countless strands, Thomas Hirschhorn suggests that we should think about the links that connect the things and facts of our existence. He seems to be reminding us that it is our duty to watch over the sequence of events, that it is there that the sense of history is born. He weaves his web the way information is transmitted, creating the knowledge of humankind, which is fragile and multiform, unverifiable and omnipresent.

In the nineties, he created gigantic collages constituted of recovered materials, packages, newspapers, magazines, small planes and electric trains. In 2000, he was awarded the prestigious Marcel Duchamp Prize.

(approx. 120 m²)

A caravan of miniature white vehicles marked with the initials of the United Nations (UN) progresses in a compact and badly ordered group. It is advancing on a rough road that is hardly visible in a black and chaotic heap of salvage materials artlessly thrown about suggesting a charred, torn up and abandoned reality. The big lorry at the lead is flying a UN flag as high in the sky as an isolated helicopter. Despite its size, compared to the immensity of the chaos, the ensign seems derisory. Yet we would like to think that these white knights of peace will provide aid and assistance to the invisible populations, who seem to be symbolically buried under the rubble. But the instability of the road holding, the messy organisation of the vehicles and especially the fact that they are all in a group are more evocative of a hasty retreat than of a triumphal arrival. Thomas Hirschhorn's installation, a detail of which we are showing here, was set up on the basis of television images of the current main armed conflicts in the world. Chechnya, Iraq, East Timor are among the many conflicts, soon forgotten by the media, that he used to form this landscape of desolation and destruction, a sort of concentrate of misfortune and absurdity. Compared to efforts of destruction, those of protection and assistance appear derisory but nonetheless testify to determination at work. Thomas Hirschhorn, a worker-artist-soldier as he likes to describe himself, thus positions himself as much as a committed artist, sensitive to the problems of his time, as outside of any ideological or artistic movement.

Like the ravaged world on which this fragile humanitarian caravan is moving forward, the successive episodes of bipolar disorder will progressively destroy the weft on which the patient's life is woven daily. Indeed, because of their intensity — and despite their total intercritical recovery — the depression and/or the mania often destroy the patient's vital bases. Whether we are evoking in manic patients their excessive spending, which might have definitely run them or their family to disaster or whether we are interested in their behaviour disorders, perceived as inappropriate at work or in their couple, we can measure the importance of the "collateral damage" that can result from the manic state. Similarly, whether we are dealing in the depressed patient with a long sick leave or a suicide attempt, the social severity of the disorder persists long after the clinical recovery of the episode has taken place. Thus, it is sometimes on an existential territory devastated by the consequences of their previous episodes that bipolar subjects move on even if they are well. It is often like the wars that Hirschhorn describes in his installation: the acting out during the manic or depressive episodes appear, when they take place, to be the fruit of "justified" decisions. Thus, the self-assurance and excitement of manic patients, which had given them the impression that their financial choices and their conquests were legitimate, or even exemplary, were the "justification" of their choices. Similarly, depressed patients, convinced by their pessimistic understanding of the world and full of the certainty of their pointlessness and helplessness, "justify" their suicidal gesture "rationally". Once the mental balance is recovered, what remains of these unshakable certainties? We understand why, once health has been recuperated, bipolar subjects often still discern, within their most immediate daily life, vestigial fragments of their pathological states. They then know they are vulnerable and understand the interest of the treatment and the need for co-operation with others, health professionals in particular. Even though it is sometimes somewhat chaotic, care makes it possible to continue moving on provided one remains grouped with the other aid providers: family, support groups and the relational network in general.

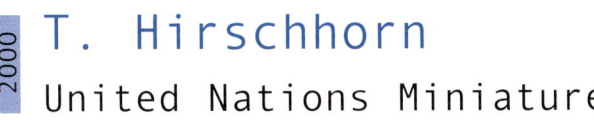

T. Hirschhorn
2000
United Nations Miniature

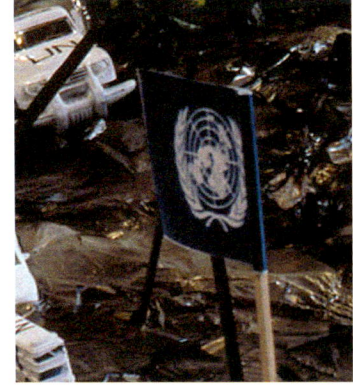

Mixed States

With simultaneous symptoms of a depressive nature and of a manic nature, mixed states were described in some of their aspects as early as the Antiquity by Aretaeus of Cappadocia, then in the early eighteenth century by Pierre-Augustin Boissier de Savages (1710-1795), William Cullen (1710-1790) and their successors.

They were not fully individualised, however, until 1896 by Emil Kraepelin within what was called at the time the Manic-depressive Psychosis (10,11). A student and close collaborator of Emil Kraepelin in Heidelberg, Wilhem Weygandt published in 1889, the year of the sixth edition of his master's famous *Textbook*, the first work in psychiatric literature exclusively devoted to mixed states. It was called *Über die Mischzustande des Manisch-Depressiven Irreseins* (On the Mixed States of Manic-Depressive Insanity). In it, is a description of the main characteristics of mixed states: *''. . . during a manic episode, the euphoria can suddenly change into a deeply depressive mood, while the other symptoms of exaltation, such as hyperkinesia and hyperactivity, distractibility and excitability, logorrhoea and flight of ideas persist; or after a month-long depression, suddenly a smile can be observed on the face of the patient and the depressive mood can change for hours or days into a high or manic mood, but without any change in psychomotor behaviour, in the inhibition or, sometimes, in the severe stupor. Less common, but actually frequent enough if observation is careful, is a temporary change in psychomotor behaviour while the affective aspects of the psychosis continue without any change; the patients remain euphoric, but the manic excitability changes into a psychomotor inhibition. Instead of tireless hyperactivity, the patients stay in bed, show slowness of movements, but no mutism. In patients with the phenomenological picture of depression with stupor, one can sometimes observe a change to mild excitability, agitation, and urge to speak lasting for hours or days, while the depressive mood continues . . . These states, very well known, but because of their short duration usually less noted, are a mix of manic and depressive episodes of circular insanity''* (17).

After a period of limbo during which mixed states were no longer considered as an autonomous entity, Himmelhoch (1976) and other North American authors, Hagop Akiskal in particular (1), showed interest in the identification of this clinical characteristic. Mixed states are henceforth fully part of the DSM-IV (6), where they are described as a remarkable clinical form of bipolar disorder.

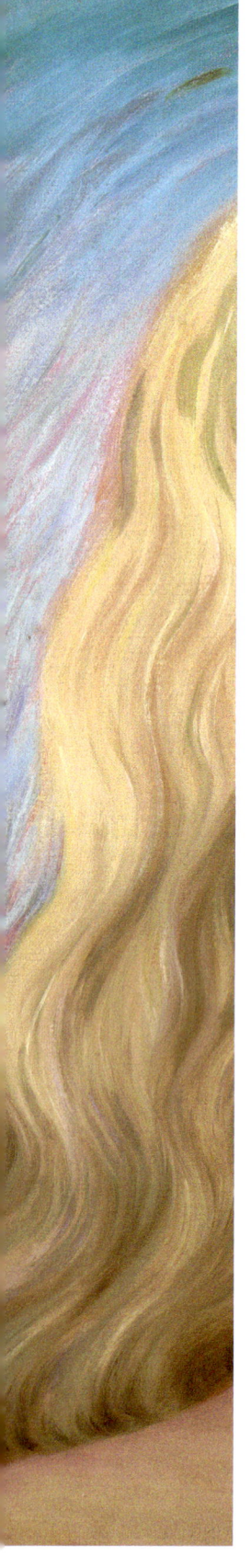

There she is, taking up all the space. She's a blonde, a blonde with heavy hair, a thick wig framing what then becomes a face: an incomplete, embryonic face… a body-face. A body with pubescent femininity, smooth and inexpressive. A head with no head, eyes with no gaze and a voiceless mouth. A woman reduced to a body, exposed and unaware of being exposed at the same time.

Yet this femininity reduced to its attributes is not attractive. It provokes discomfort and embarrassment, an effect accentuated by the pastel, almost insipid background with fuzzy contours. This headless woman is not someone that can be spoken with, she is no longer even a woman. All that is left of her is this bulging body with too much flesh, the headless object of an unrequited desire that excluded her from herself.

During manic states, an erotisation of contacts is often observed. As much the body as the mind is used to seduce in a staging that underscores the social features of a caricatured love relationship. Ideally, a love relationship is built on the basis of reciprocity, where both attempt to convey to each other the essence of their singularity and their difference. Manic patients, instead, try to seduce by using seduction attributes that are consensually acknowledged by the social group. In the same way that they stage their body, they invest other persons not so much for themselves as because in their eyes they display an analogous array of desirability codes. In Magritte's painting, the blond hair and the smooth body with budding feminine forms offered for others to see juxtapose three archetypal canons of femininity. The essential is missing: the singularity of the one who is exhibiting them, that is, her head, her gaze, her speech.

1945 René Magritte
The Rape

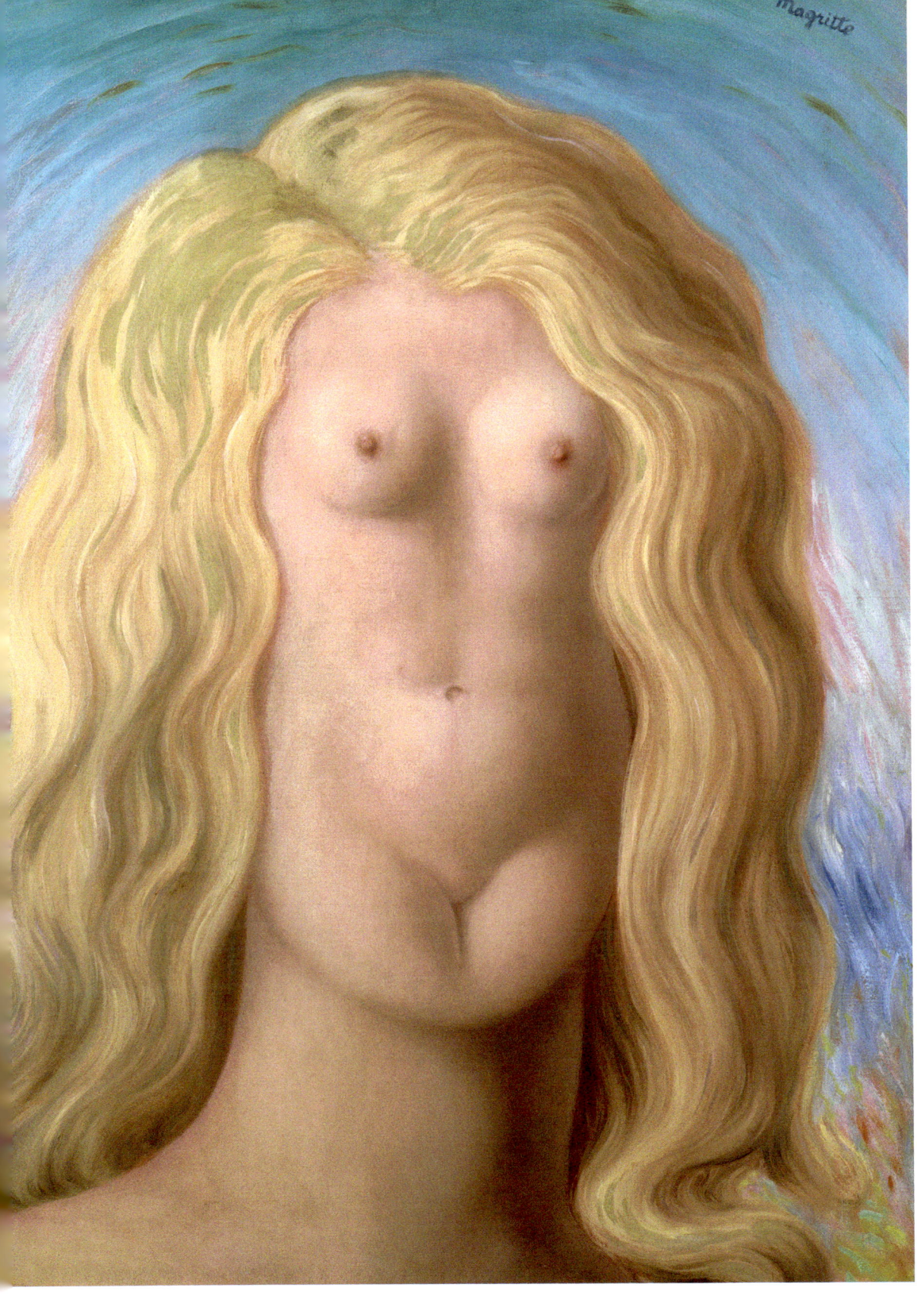

An unobtrusive man and a true Mister Nobody in his life, the Belgian surrealist painter, **René Magritte** (1898-1967) was, in his art, a master of surprises and a prince of the absurd. Falsely ingenuous, his painting, associating hyperrealism and incongruities, is amongst the most subversive there is. It was not so much beings and objects that Magritte was interested in as the way that they related to one another. Specializing in a sort of tongue-in-cheek humour, he played with reality by constantly raising doubts as to the identity of what he represented. His paintings are enigmas or traps that are confusing and can provoke in the viewer a feeling of uneasiness, or even of anguish.

(65.3 x 50.4 cm)

58

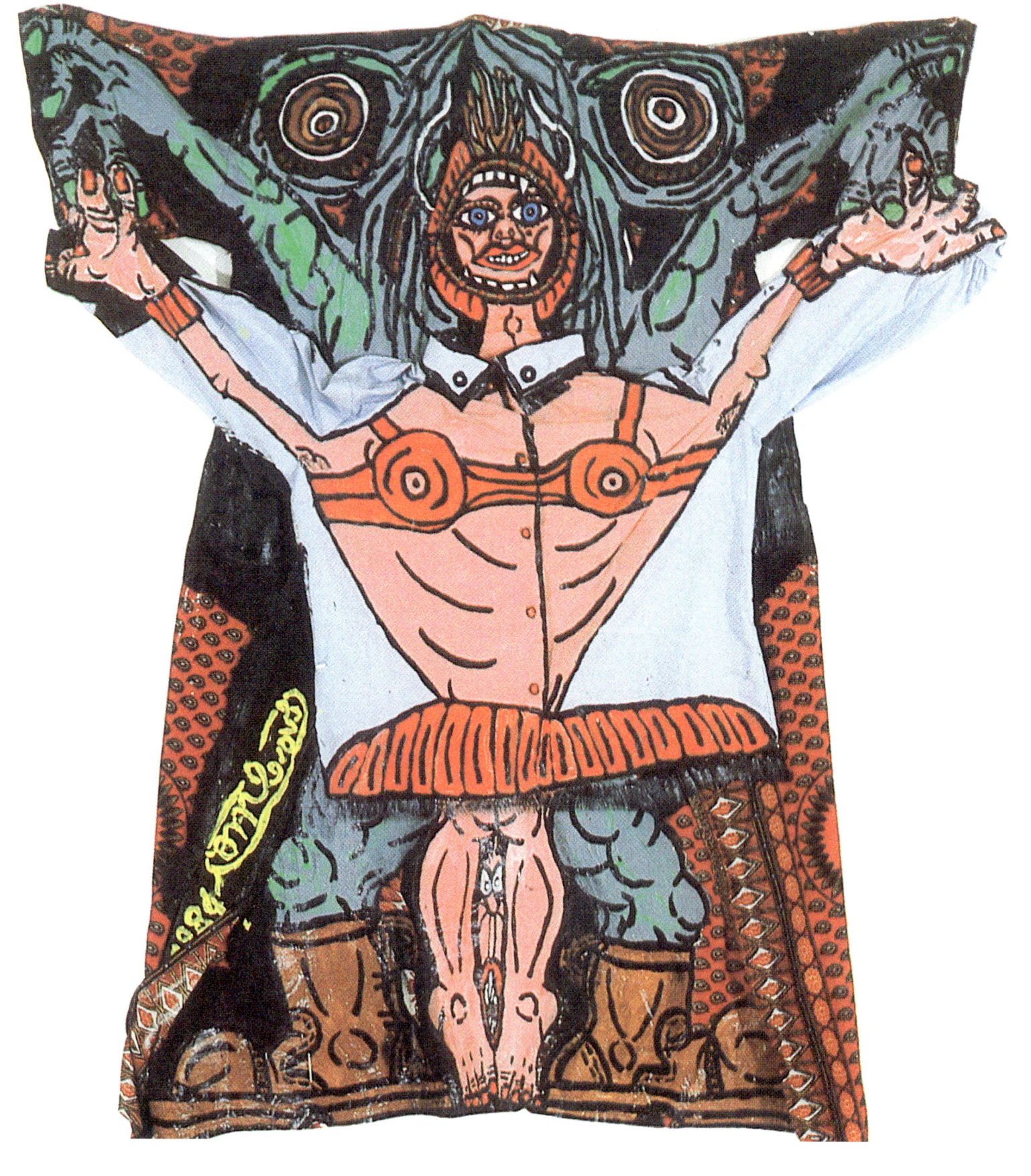

— DISTRESS — TRAVESTY — DEMONSTRATIVE — DISTRESS — TRAVESTY — DEMONSTRATIVE — DISTRESS — TRAVESTY —

The central character, arms wide open, bursts into our visual field. Is he crucified? we wonder. Is he calling us? His huge blue eyes are looking beyond us. His neck is sticking out of a shirt that is too large, painted in trompe-l'oeil. The short red skirt and the hollow bra in the centre, on a broad and brawny torso, suggest a caricature of travesty. At the extremity of his slender arms, the enormous hands seem not to belong to him anymore. We then discover, in the middle distance, a greenish monster with a lumpy body, staring at us, wild-eyed. Its wide-open mouth encloses the head of the central character, who is thus inside and outside at the same time. If we continue to explore, we distinguish a third character, his face jammed between the first one's legs. What are all these interlocked beings looking at?

This heterogeneous fitting together of representations, each with a strong power of suggestion (crucifixion, travesty, science-fiction), has a paradoxical unity. The peculiar fantasy displayed by patients in a manic phase is so inseparable from their immediate experience that it does not evoke a masquerade. Nonetheless, like the central character of the painting who, when observed, becomes one amongst others, the patient's very demonstrative immediate appearance loses its panache in an interview and shows the distress behind it.

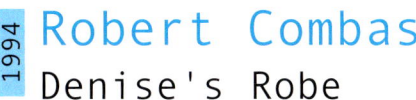

Robert Combas
Denise's Robe

1994

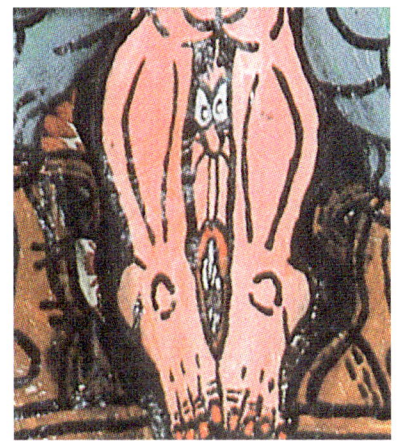

Robert Combas was born in Lyons in 1957. His painting takes its inspiration from rock music, which he likes, from popular images, from children's books or schoolbooks. He is the creator of the "Figuration Libre" of the eighties, a painting style that is "fun, funny and relaxed". A form of expressionism that he also defines as "an experiment towards a universal language".

He likes using the greatest variety of material, clothes in particular, which he collects and paints, as for the robe and the shirt in this work.

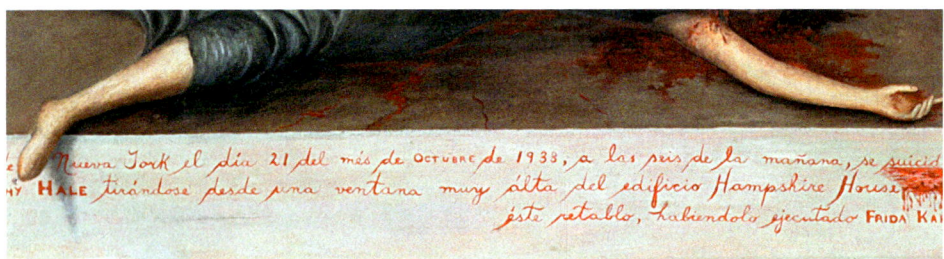

Frida Kahlo
1939
The Suicide of Dorothy Hale

Here, the frame does not contain, it is part of the painting. Its absence takes into infinity the feathery space of a reality to which the dead woman no longer belongs. Although she is already on the ground, like a broken doll whose foot seems to be outside of the painting, she continues to fall. Frida Kahlo has stacked around a central axis a massive, isolated and concentrationary building, an Icarus-angel with a frozen expression and the body of a woman lying on the ground in a classic draped dress. The caption that can be distinguished at the bottom of the painting and which seems to have been written with the dead woman's blood, makes one think of a naturalist's scholarly comment. Underneath, the frame is bare and stained with blood. Such precision and the realism of the representation underscore the impression of a reality with no transcendence. We are helpless before the fall and in the after event of death at the same time.

Although suicide frequently conveys, in the familiar circles, the duality of the horror of the gesture and the powerlessness to go back in time, it is often considered by the depressed patient as an attempt to escape from the suffering of his illness. Prisoners of depression, constrained to sadness and to a pejorative cognitive treatment of the world that surrounds them, depressed patients sometimes believe to have found in suicide a solution that would still depend on them in a world where they perceive no way out. Although resulting from pathological mechanisms independent of their will, the pejorative perception of the world possesses such realism that it invades depressed patients, for whom the world then appears as completely intolerable. They are subsequently tempted to jump out of the window of an excessively constrained reality.

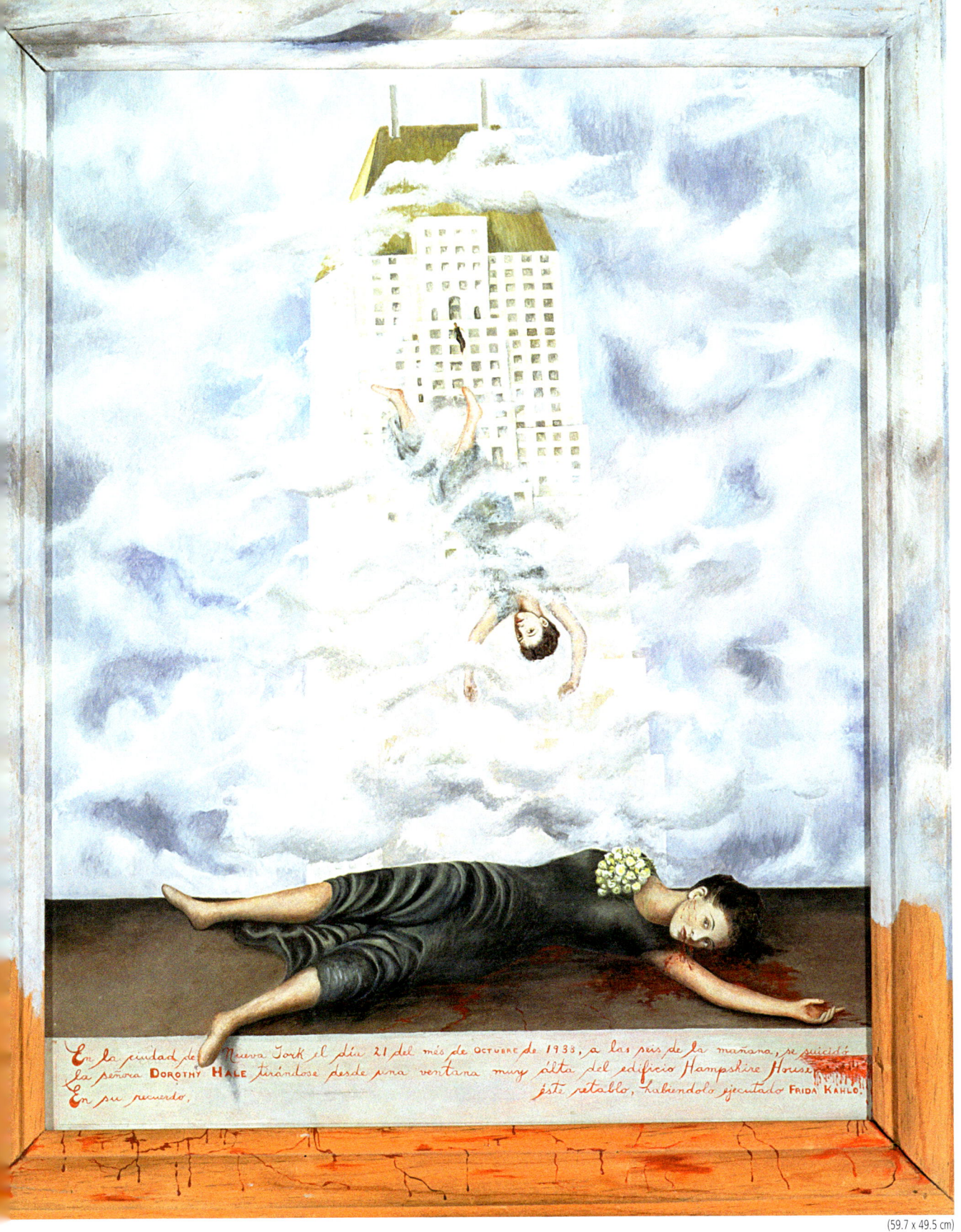

(59.7 x 49.5 cm)

The work of the Mexican **Frida Kahlo** (1910-1954) is entirely dominated by suffering. In her numerous self-portraits – she produced more than seventy – this young woman of singular beauty staged her body tortured by polio and the results of a serious bus accident, sometimes donning it with the most flamboyant traditional clothes of her country, sometimes showing it naked, corseted or torn apart.

In this work, Frida Kahlo was inspired by an actual news item, which she relates in the lower part of the painting:

"In New York City on the 21st of October 1938, at 6:00 in the morning, Dorothy Hale committed suicide by throwing herself from a very high window in the Hampshire House. In her memory […], this *retablo* was executed by Frida Kahlo".

1964 Sempé — Sit!

At the bottom of a nearly blank page, waves are breaking in a frieze pattern. They are dashing in from the right in anthropomorphous volutes, more amused than dangerous, with their hair of crest and foam. Hokusai comes to mind, of course, with his famous wave. As they come closer to the beach, the swells sober down and the billows turn into pointy wavelets, then into innocuous ripples. The ocean reaches the feet of an incongruous character: too small, too urban, too debonair. He is the archetype of the average Frenchman and you laugh when you read, in very small print, the order that he utters: "Sit!". The humour comes from the lack of proportion between the indomitable immensity of the ocean spread all over the page, and this small, insignificant fellow, standing there, claiming with calm assurance to command Nature.

Our character seems not to have the slightest doubt. Against all evidence — since he very obviously cannot tame the ocean — he pronounces the imperious injunction: "Sit!" Omnipotence or unconsciousness? Perhaps a bit of both. The megalomania of patients in a manic state, though it often has more arrogance than that of Sempé's tiny gentleman, has, however, many points in common with it. Their common megalomania contains an underestimation of the situation and of the conspicuous signs of a challenge, at the same time that they often seem to be part of a grandiloquent production. Like Sempé's character, manic patients provoke laughter and are intriguing at the same time: the humour comes as much from the naïve assurance that they display as from the derisory or disproportionate nature of the task that they assign themselves. All at once worried, because they feel fragile, greedy for recognition, because they are afraid not to be taken seriously, and driven by the constantly flowing surge of ideas and emotions, manic patients, although they are sometimes amusing, have neither the tenacity of a paranoiac patient nor the decision-maker's assurance when they claim that they wish to undertake something. They run in order not to fall.

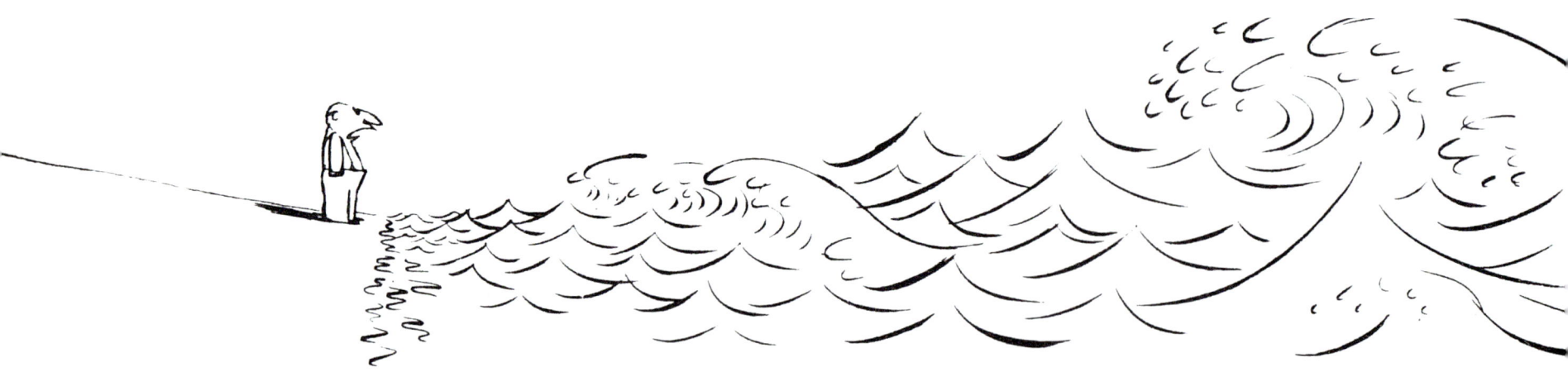

– *Couché !*
– *Sit !*

— MEGALOMANIA — HUMOUR — UNAWARENESS — MEGALOMANIA — HUMOUR — UNAWARENESS — MEGALOMANIA — HUMOU

The French comic artist **Jean-Jacques Sempé** was born on 17 August 1932 in Bordeaux. Self-educated, he had had his drawings published in several newspapers when he met René Goscinny, in 1954, with whom he invented, four years later, a small character who was to make them famous the world over: Le petit Nicolas – Little Nicolas. Since then, he has never stopped publishing: from 1962 to today, from Rien n'est simple – Nothing is simple – to Beau Temps – Good weather – about thirty books in all. At the same time, he has continued to contribute to many magazines – Paris-Match, Punch, L'Express – and has made at least sixty covers for the New Yorker. His delicate, subtle and allusive humour with a remarkable sense of the derisory characterises all his work. His drawings propose a tenderly ironic vision of our shortcomings and of the shortcomings of the world.

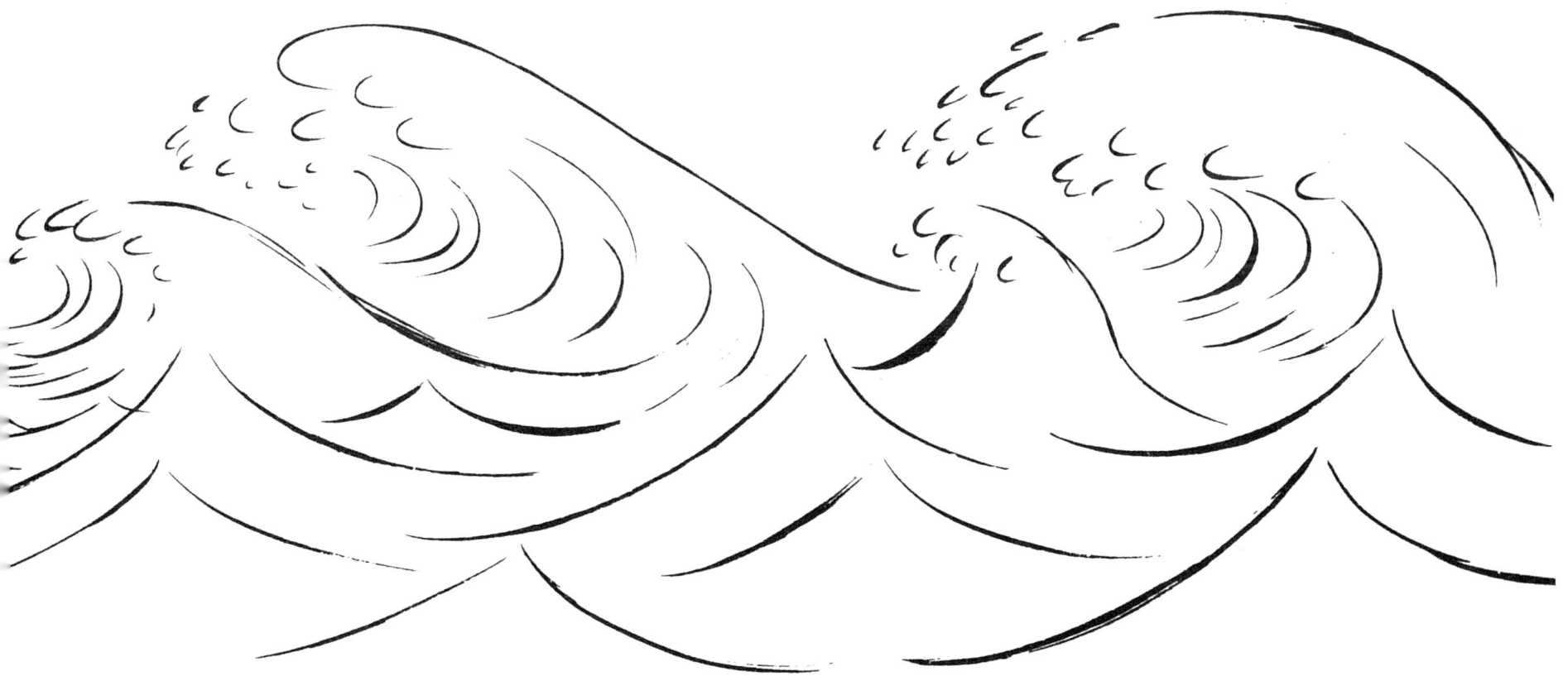

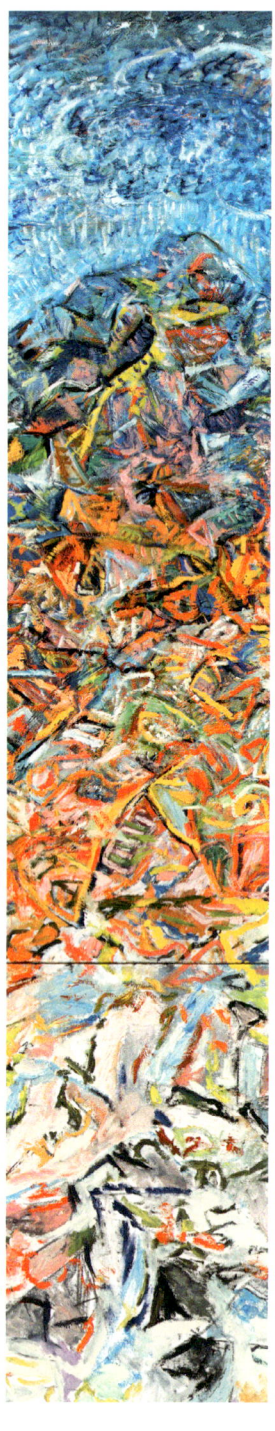

A landfill stands before our eyes like a gaudy pyramid. Inexorably, almost peacefully, it fills up the steamy blue of a sky of clouds and foam. Colourful packages, roughly crumpled paper, the leftovers of an appearance and consumption society, have piled up to form this enormous, composite and empty mound. Who is the craftsman of this occurrence? An individual as unlikely in his size as in his clothing: a suit, town shoes and a ridiculously small hat. He is carrying a voluminous ball without the slightest effort. Will it break up and spread over the pile, as suggested by its colour, or will it roll down the other side once it is on top? We will never know, despite the title of the painting, The Idleness of Sisyphus, which refers to the useless labour, forever started over, of the hero of ancient times who was punished by the gods. The character's impassive face, his closed eyes and his half smile suggest the mechanical repetition of his ascent. No weariness, no desire – everything is happening as if the achievement of this task was self-evident. The mountain, although largely composed of vacuum, will not be packed down with time. Indeed, in the lower panel, the faded rubbish has kept its original volume.

One of the features of bipolar disorder is the repetition of the manic or depressive episodes. Clinical experience and studies have shown that life events with a powerful emotional charge only trigger relapses at the beginning of the disorder. After that, failing treatment, the disorder reappears according to inexorable cycles, in the image of the unflappable and almost automatic climb of Sandro Chia's character. As symbolised by the mountain thus constituted, the patient's life, when he recovers his health, remains unfailingly cluttered by the consequences of the succession of past episodes. Like the voluminous but empty objects presented in the mountain, episodes of the disorder take up all the space when they express themselves but appear not to have existed when they have stopped, and yet their presence, like these packages that will never be packed down, progressively erode the healthy person's space.

Sandro Chia
1981
The Idleness of Sisyphus

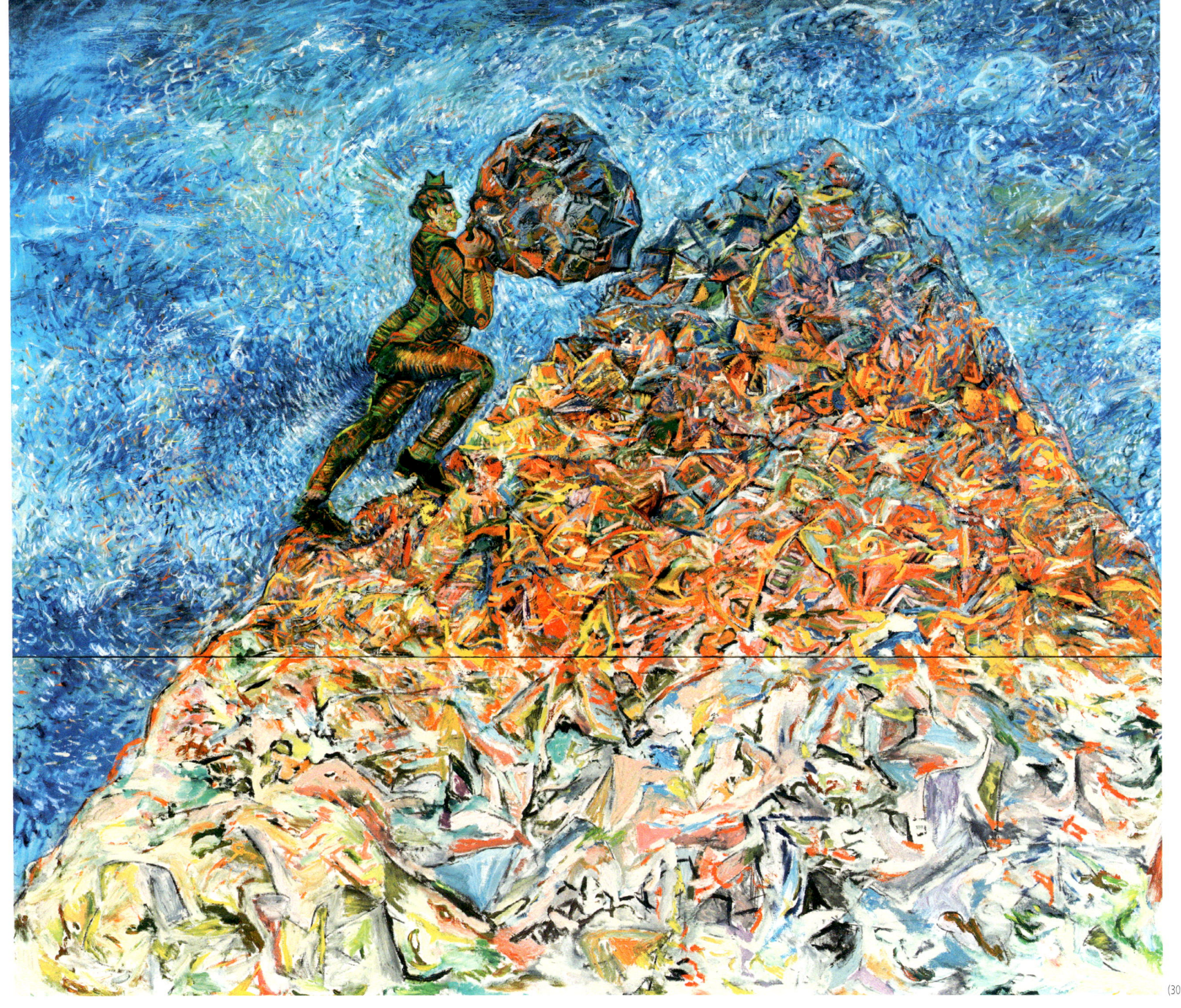

(309.9 x 386.7 cm)

*Painter, lithographer, sculptor and traveller, **Sandro Chia**, who was born in Florence in 1946, lives today between Rome, New York and Montalcino, Italy. In the seventies, he was one of the prominent figures of the Italian Transavantguardia, which undertook to take up with a certain form of painting again: figuration and narration. With other painters of his generation, he reappropriated the traditional images and myths of his country by using a multitude of pictorial languages, from Neo-Mannerism to Neo-Expressionism, including Fauvism and Symbolism.*

Key Data on Bipolarity

DEFINITIONS

Bipolar disorder I: diagnosis can be established from a single manic episode. In the majority of cases, Bipolar Patients I who have expressed one or several manic episodes have also presented one or several clear depressive episodes at another moment of their clinical history.

Bipolar disorder II: diagnosis can be established when there has been at least one hypomaniac episode (an attenuated form of mania featuring mainly an elevated mood resulting most often from an increase in energy and self-confidence) and a clear depressive episode.

Mixed State: clinical state during which the patient presents signs of mania and depression concomitantly. Suicide risk is greater during this state.

Psychotic features (delusion, hallucinations)
They are found in 50% of mania cases.
They are rarer in depression and are seen mainly in its severe forms

DSM-IV (Diagnostic and Statistical Manual for Mental Disorders, 4th edition)
Classification of mental disorders published by the American Association of Psychiatry.

CIM-10 (International Classification of Mental Diseases and Behavioural Comportment, 10th edition)
Classification of mental disorders published by the World Health Organisation.

INCIDENCE
(The differences in percentage values correspond on the one hand to the classification – DSM or CIM – chosen for the studies and on the other hand to the more-or-less inclusive interpretation of the psychological manifestations of the persons examined by the raters).

Bipolar I: 0.5% to 1% of the general population presents the symptoms necessary for establishing a diagnosis of Bipolar Disorder I.

Bipolar II: 0.4% to 11% of the general population present the symptoms necessary for establishing a diagnosis of Bipolar Disorder II.

Distribution by gender: identical incidence for both genders.

Maximum incidence peak for the first episode of the disorder: age 15 to 25. There have been descriptions of very early beginnings in children (under 10 years old) or of first episodes after age 80, but these are very rare possibilities.

GENETICS
Family studies:
In a family, when one of the members is affected by bipolar disorder, the chances that another member of this family should be affected are about 6%, whereas they are about 0.5% amongst the population in general.
The risk of being affected by the disorder is all the greater that the family member has a severe form of it.
The current studies show that – as opposed to other mental disorders – the environment or other factors influencing the development of the central nervous system have little influence on the appearance of bipolar disorder.

Studies on twins:
Identical twins (monozygotic): the second twin presents the criteria of the disorder in 60% of cases where the first is affected.
Fraternal twins (dizygotic): the second twin presents the criteria of the disorder in 14% of cases where the first is affected.

Genes involved:
Several genes are involved in the development of bipolar disorder.

BIOLOGY
Dopamine (neurotransmitter present in some of the synapses of the central nervous system; it is involved in movement, emotion, attention, sense-organ activity and in the regulation of certain hormones). The manic state is associated with an increase of dopamine consumption by the brain, a comparable situation to that resulting from having taken amphetamines, which induce symptoms very similar to those of the manic state. This increase in dopamine consumption adequately explains the agitation, the absence of need for sleep, the increase in sexuality and the difficulties that manic patients show in fixing their attention. But the increase in dopamine activity cannot alone explain the set of symptoms in patients in a manic state and even less the bipolar disorder in general.

Other brain neurotransmitters:
They are moderately or not involved in bipolar disorder.

References (8,9)

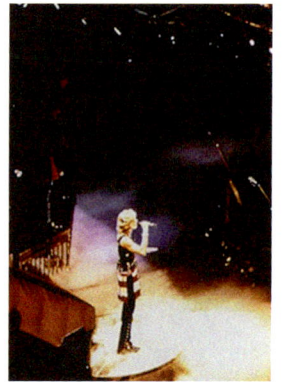

Andreas Gursky
Madonna I
2001

Dots of light, sometimes coloured like confetti, are haphazardly suspended against a black background, which they occupy completely. Although it is immense, Gursky's photo seems to have caught no more than the fragment of a colossal crowd. The title informs us that these shimmering speckles reflect the incalculable spectators – or perhaps only part of them – come to watch the performer Madonna for one of her series of shows in Los Angeles in 2001. Have they switched on their lighters all together, in communion with the singer, or is this an effect of camera flashes or of sweeping spotlights with a gigantic range? We will never know. Moving quickly on from an analysis of the details, we take a broader look, intrigued by the dark curve in the centre, by the metallic structures, then by the irregular splashes of warmer-coloured light. These form a sort of stretched-out arc erected before the singer, whom we then discover off centre and seeming to have been placed that way on the stage. We then take a fresh start and begin to look for anecdotal elements: we try to scrutinise the picture for anything that would allow us to grasp the specificity of that evening in Los Angeles. Instead, we only wander in search of some kind of unity on this moving and luminous matter made of distant and impersonal living beings: the photographer's partial and almost frontal framing does not allow us to catch a general view of the concert. The both precise and distant nature of this picture, completely realistic and unreal at the same time, comes from the fact that Andreas Gursky reconstructed this photograph from about 15 negatives of shots taken on different days, at about the same moment of the finale of Madonna's concert. With computer technology, he touched up certain parts, sometimes pixel by pixel, to show the quintessence of this event but also to record it outside of time. In seizing emblematic places of our contemporary society, Gursky seeks to show that it is made of multitude and anonymity, of immediate accession to its most minute parts but at the same time impossible to grasp in its totality.

Some of the mental processes of the manic patient are similar to our constant movements as we look at this photograph. Continuously going from the analysis of some minute detail to that of the immense without ever being able to grasp in their totality unity and true reality – in the sense of the reality where one is able to act – the manic patient is caught up in an intellectual and sensory, almost hypnotic activity. The world as the patient perceives it is thus constituted by an infinitely rich and iridescent reality that can however never be completely grasped in its unity. Recomposed because of the excessive association of ideas and emotions that are connected with it, the reality on which manic patients found their analysis and their decisions has thus often lost the qualities it needs for its pragmatic use. The decisions made, often unrealistic, therefore result from a shortage in the sense of the unity and the context of the experienced situation. Just as the figure of Madonna – central to understanding the photo – is off centre and hieratic, the key element of the experienced situation that would allow it to be understood becomes marginal in the manic patient's perception. The result is the discrepancy and agitation characteristic of the disorder. The medicinal and psychotherapeutic treatment then aims to help the patient break out of this indistinction, made of signifiers that are far too many and at the same time not enough to be efficient. Gursky's approach, although it is close to a manic patient's, is creative insofar as it aims to depict the shortcomings of a contemporary world made of mass movements and appearances, in which the subject remains alone in the crowd. On the other hand, although bipolar patients can in some cases be creative, the manic state is never the period when they create.

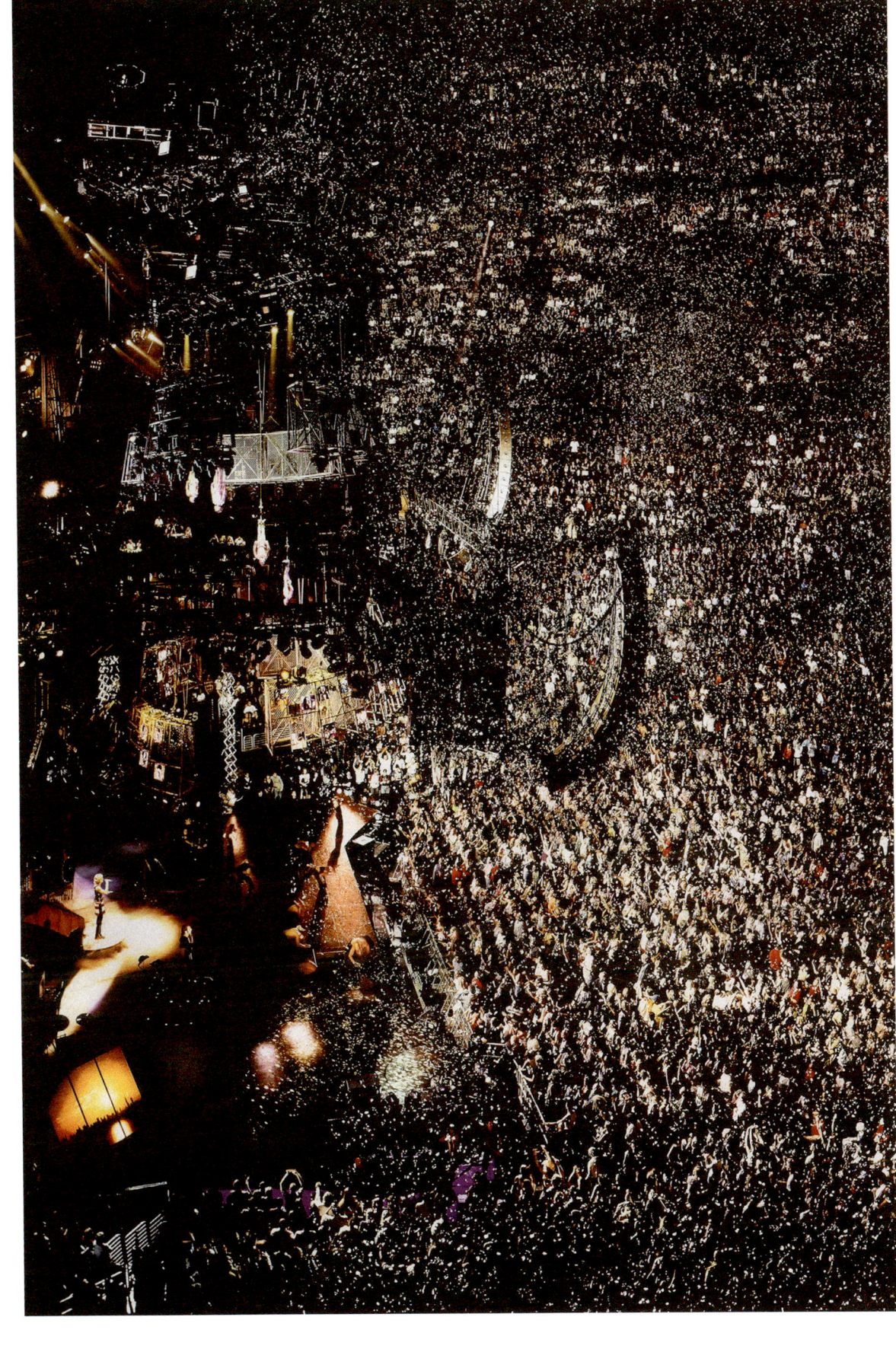

*The German photographer **Andreas Gursky** was born in 1955. He shows people seen from a great distance, like confetti, stardust or ants inside the rooms and tunnels they have built for themselves in their anthill. Gursky opposes the unity of a crowd and the multiplicity of its subjects, the gigantic and the infinitely small, the impersonal and the personal. He dramatizes a world that never moves on from the project stage. As a result, something "sounds wrong". Gursky's places are impossible places, closer to sensations than to reality.*

Gursky marks an absolute distance with regard to reality, trying thus to offer a new, crushing vision of it, which accentuates the fragility or emptiness of man, of the individual facing multiplicity.

His work has been presented at the Pompidou Centre and the New York Museum of Modern Art.

(275 x 200 cm)

70

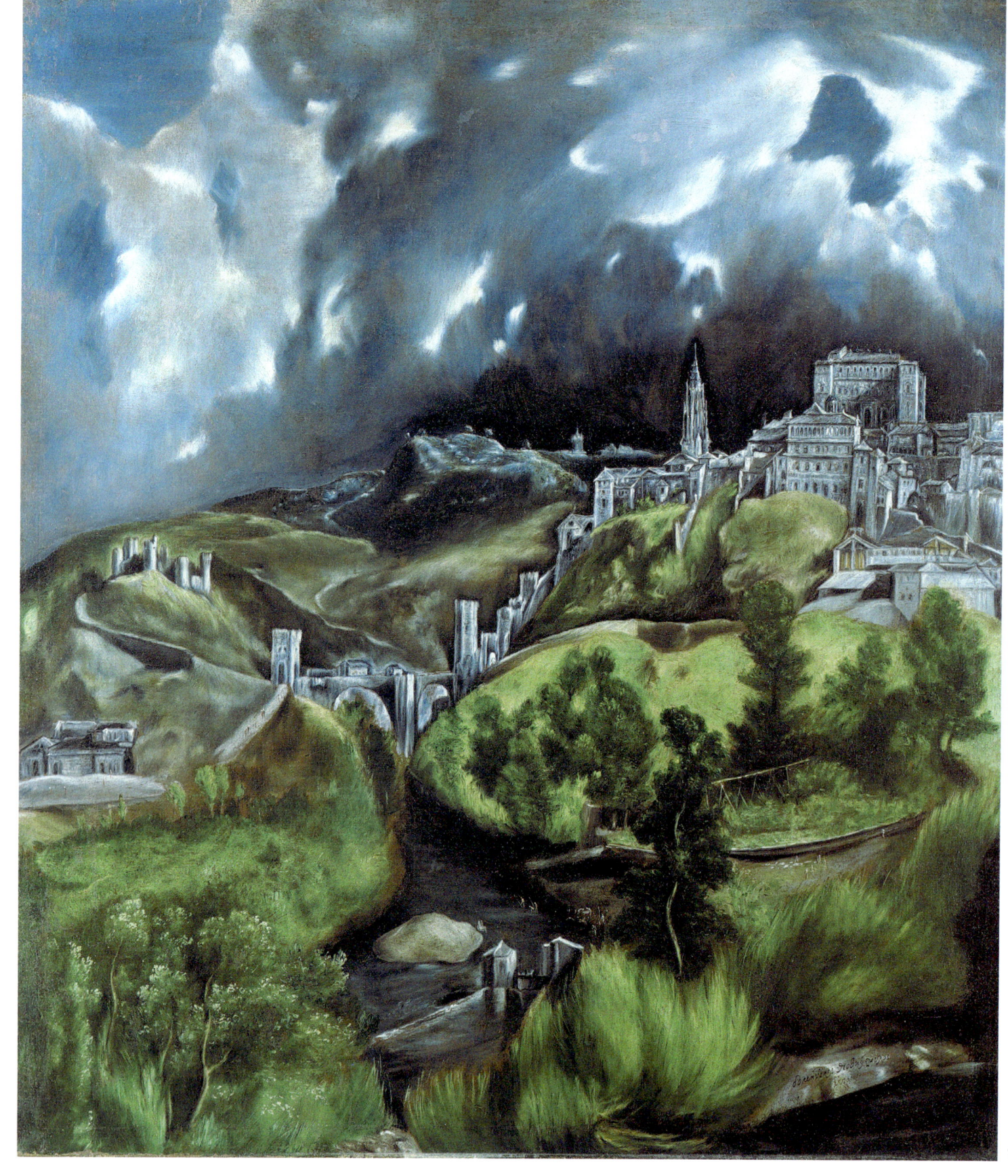

(121.3 x 108.6 cm)

— HINDERED — WITHOUT REST — VIOLENCE OF REALITY — HINDERED — WITHOUT REST — VIOLENCE OF REALITY — HINDER

El Greco
View of Toledo
1597

At the right of the painting stands a grey city, compact and mineral. It rules over an unlikely landscape portioned into uninviting plots. The acid-green countryside, built up like a progression of barriers, forms a first rampart followed by an all but derisory one made of stone, set in the middle distance. Beyond the border of the fortified bridge lies an arid, barren area. The path drawn into it loses itself in the blackness of the sky. It seems to prolong the river in the foreground, the dark waters of which have been made impassable by the rocks and constructions. This succession of natural and human obstacles lead one's gaze, in stages, towards the patch of sky torn into the mass of black clouds concentrated over the city. Will the storm finally break?

The inner world of melancholic patients, as in El Greco's painting, is made of obstructed spaces. As far as they can see, there seems to be no exit from these territories, all closed up unto themselves, to a more peaceful place where they might be able to rest and then go elsewhere. Their pain is not any more likely to find comfort in Nature than in the city of men. The foreknowledge that they believe to have of the world to its very last details, as if they were standing in a light similar to the one illuminating The Greek's landscape, corroborates their evidence that any effort is useless. In some cases, when the struggle seems hopeless and disaster imminent, the patient can long for death as the ultimate recourse. Once the episode is treated and overcome, patients recover the freedom to walk in the world's landscape.

*Cretan-born, Domenikos Theotokopoulos (1541-1614) went into posterity as **El Greco** Spanish painter. Marked first by the Greco-Byzantine influence of his native Crete, he went on to train in Rome. At age 35, he started out for Castile where he tried to obtain the favours of the powerful King Philip II of Spain, before finally settling in Toledo, where he found generous patronage. This view of the former imperial city is the only known landscape of the painter, otherwise famous for the mannerism of his long-drawn-out bodies, the expressionism of the movements of his characters, the acidity of his colouration and his tendency to abstraction in his treatment of volumes.*

72

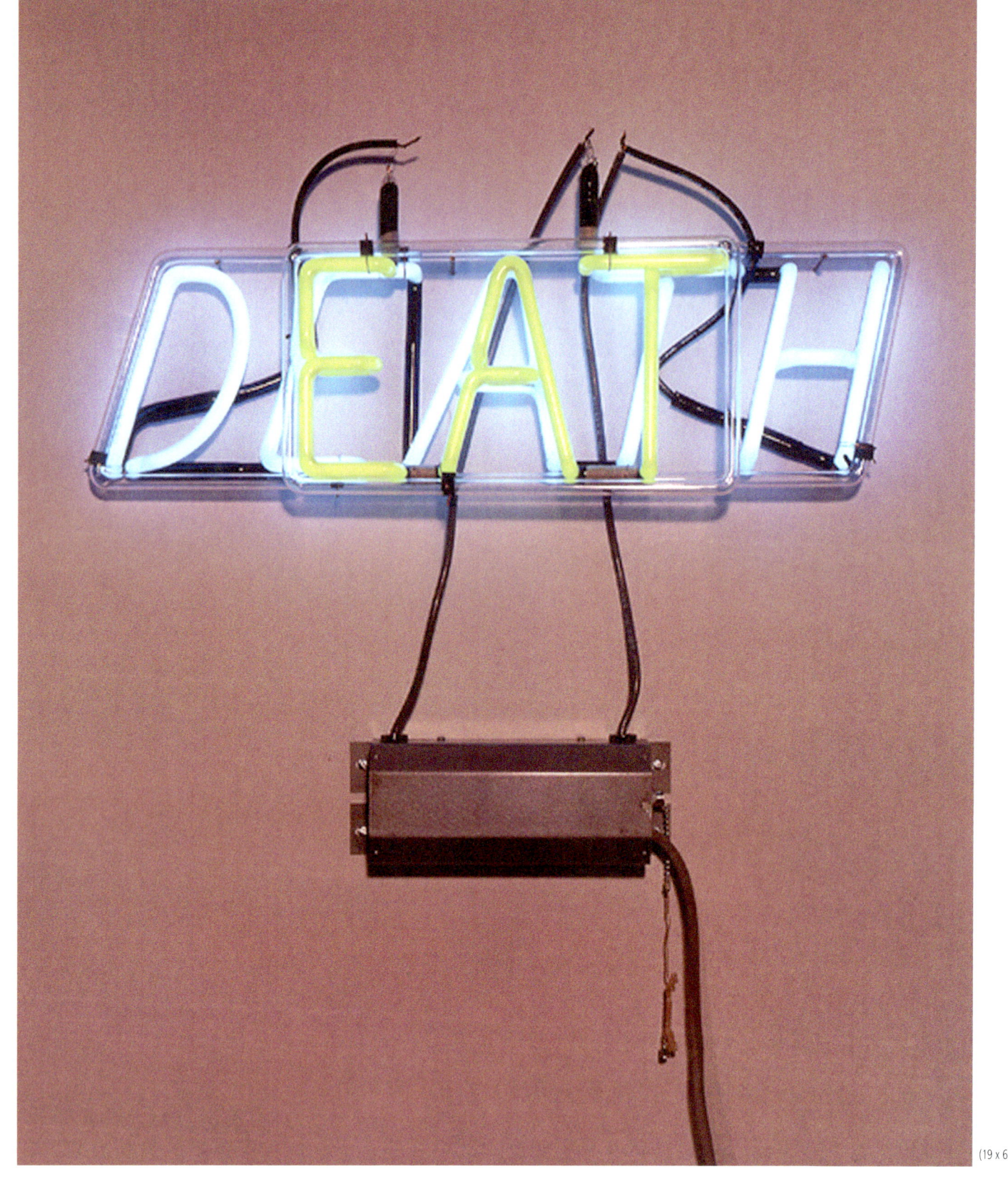

(19 x 64 x 15 cm)

ORRHOEA — POLYSEMY — ISOLATION — LOGORRHOEA — POLYSEMY — ISOLATION — LOGORRHOEA — POLYSEMY — ISOLA

In a frame of translucent pipes connected to conspicuously visible electric wiring, the two words EAT and DEATH are superimposed where their three common letters meet: E, A and T. One yellow, one blue, they light up in turn. The uppercase letters– straight for EAT and in italics for DEATH – blink endlessly in monotonous succession. They evoke as much the circularity of the life-food/death couple as its implacable and anonymous repetition. The urban solitude of the neon lights, the pressure of life and the dehumanisation of daily life, the ephemeral precariousness of words and the duplicity of meaning are concentrated in what can appear to constitute no more than an innocent luminous gadget.

In the manic patient, words succeed one another incessantly, vividly colourful, bumping into one another rather than finding their articulation. In spite of their iridescent and inventive appearance, the words are constrained into a system of implacable repetition. They pile up and are juxtaposed, all set – for some brilliant play on words, for some unique association – to lose the logical progression by which they are articulated. The communication function of language thus disappears to the benefit of a glimmer on the surface. Such logorrhoea, paying little attention to the presence and responses of other persons, progressively isolates manic patients from their fellow citizens, who become weary of the uninterrupted and often aggressive stream of words. If we listen carefully to the terms that are employed, to the sometimes unusual way in which they are used, to their polysemy, we can infer the immense solitude, or even despair of the speaker through the avalanche of words.

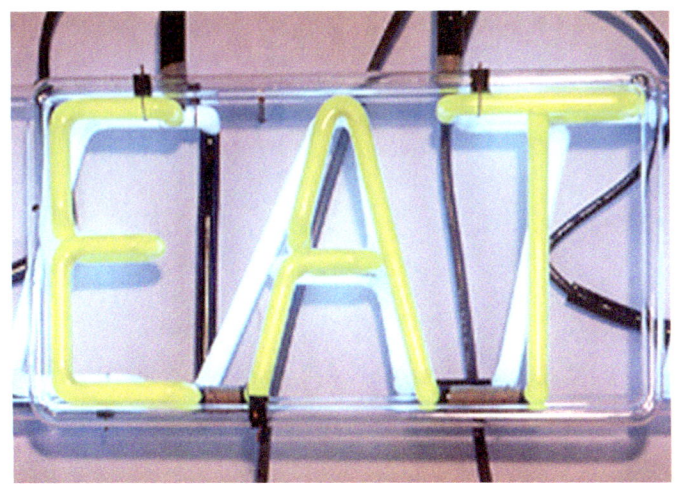

Born in Fort Wayne, Indiana, in 1941, **Bruce Nauman** *attended the University of California at Davis. He has already had many solo exhibitions in New York, Zurich, Basel and at the Pompidou Centre in Paris. It may be reality that Bruce Nauman is seeking, or helping us to seek. Close to Body Art of the early sixties, his immediate subject was his own body or his travels. His approach then developed to the creation of architectural installations. In his installation "Raw Materials", Bruce Nauman staged the same approach as in Eat/Death when he shot in an exaggeratedly narrow frame a face repeating the same sentence indefinitely, this absurd repetition thus depriving it of all its meaning. Similarly, in another of his installations (Live-taped Video Corridor), a video surveillance system placed behind the visitor gave him the impression that he was moving away as he came closer to the control monitor.*

Bruce Nauman
1972 EAT/DEATH

Bipolarity and Society?

To understand the psychology of individuals, two complementary approaches are usually referred to.

The first studies thoughts, emotions and behaviour as experiences by the subjects. Thus, even though the content of our thoughts, the nature of our emotions or the components of our behaviour can be classified under major categories, the way each of us experiences them is unique: no one other than ourselves experiences them at the same moment or in our place. This perspective is thus interested in the psychology of persons considered in their singularity and their uniqueness.

The second approach considers that individuals cannot be understood outside of the society in which they live. Indeed, language, beliefs and social habits are pre-existent to individuals. As it is impossible for individuals to develop alone, without at least referring to their family, they are immersed from their birth onwards in a socio-cultural context by which they are deeply permeated. Language is an example of the fact that there are social codes that do not depend on us and yet thanks to which we can assert our singularity. To be able to say "I", we need to have assimilated not only language but also a large number of social communication codes. Similarly, our family precedes us and, with it, a host of values, habits and beliefs that we progressively make our own without our even realizing it.

Thus, like the two – inseparable – sides of the same coin, one's psychological identity is at the same time the fruit of one's uniqueness and the product of the socio-cultural group from which one comes.

A number of psychiatrists and psychologists have taken an interest in the "social side" of mental patients when analysing their symptoms. They have sought to understand whether their psychological manifestations might reflect the suffering of their social individuality. Such authors have themselves supported this type of analysis with sociological theories.

We shall single out two of these theories for a simplified description of them.
The first sociological theory is derived from structuralism. For structuralists and their successors (Claude Levi-Strauss (13) or Pierre Bourdieu (5)), social processes are the outcome of fundamental structures that are in most cases invisible. These structures condition social organisation as a whole, generating a large numbers of practices and beliefs. These latter, applied to the individuals who make up society, will fashion them and condition some of their reactions. Having become practically automatic (habitus), these reactions are not perceived as having been learned.
The second theory, on which antipsychiatry was largely founded, postulates that there are dominant frames of reference in our societies, usually those of a minority group. Being hegemonic, this value system is imposed on the rest of the social group, generating frustration and suffering. Mentioned by these authors to illustrate the arbitrary nature of the dominant group's norms are the limits between normality and mental illness, which vary according to the society.

Grounding themselves on this approach, some authors have proposed a "sociological" analysis of the symptoms of mental illnesses. These latter would not, then, be the exclusive expression of a disorder having its source in the biology of the brain, education, the environment or childhood traumas. The symptoms would be a reflection of the constraints or the suffering of the societies in which the patients live. According to this analysis, some individuals can be made ill by excessive social pressure. Others' pathology could be understood as an attempt to escape unbearable environmental constraints through madness. Finally, through their symptoms, other sick persons would be amplifying – as a loudspeaker would do – the "illness" of the society in which they live.

Alluring and sometimes relevant, these models are difficult to handle because they are also the result of theories in which a significant part is arbitrary for the same reason as the models that they criticise. Their shortcoming is that they elude the importance of the biological constraints to which we are all submitted, including how our brain and our thinking work. These models also exaggerate the malleability of individuals because they postulate that their psychology is mainly the result of their assimilation of the social group's constraints to the detriment of their personal opinions. Finally, they refer to fixed social models, submitted to unchangeable laws, which is obviously not what is shown by the evolution of social groups.

Mania and Society

The increase in the number of persons in the past few years having psychological and behavioural manifestations reminiscent of bipolar disorder without actually including all the criteria of the illness led us to raise the question: Is the contemporary world bipolar?
To answer this question, we tried to consider it as a game, a game of similarities. We decided to take some of the features of bipolar disorder and examined in parallel the behaviour and the values of our contemporary world in order to identify to what extent it offers an analogy with bipolar features. To facilitate our game, we reduced our analysis to three of the major manifestations of bipolar disorder: mania, depression and recurrence. We then assigned qualities to each of these manifestations, such as for example speed for mania or solitude for depression. As we can see, it is the qualities and not the symptoms themselves – which would make no sense – that we will compare to the behaviour and the values of our contemporary society.

We selected for mania such qualities as speed, timelessness, the need for movement and the importance of change. Other points in common between contemporary values and mania should be underscored. We can mention the interest shown in our society to anything that is extreme, the attention given to appearance and the importance granted to action, often considered as preferable to pure thinking. We could also highlight the general environment of our societies, in which, as with the manic patient, the saturation of information channels scrambles all the messages, such that none of them is distinct from the background noise. Thus, our Western society's dreams and illusions are built – as with the manic patient – on fad and the belief, with no perspective, in a world in which all commodities could be grasped in the same instant. A world in which we believe we are moving more quickly by the moment, with less constraints, where we imagine we are flirting daily with the extreme limits of reality.

Contemporary art testifies to the manic nature of our society in its recourse to sophisticated technology enabling instantaneous or very spectacular performances. It reflects the acceleration of time in its installations or its ephemeral performances. Its challenging, enigmatic aspect over-informs us at the same time that it leaves us with no message. Whether it is about showing – through a process of accumulation pushed to the extreme – the consumerist excesses of our society as with Arman, or about saturating viewers with information when they are looking at a multitude of video monitors in which different images are streaming by, the contemporary artistic approach is unquestionably evocative of some of the manic aspects of our contemporary world.

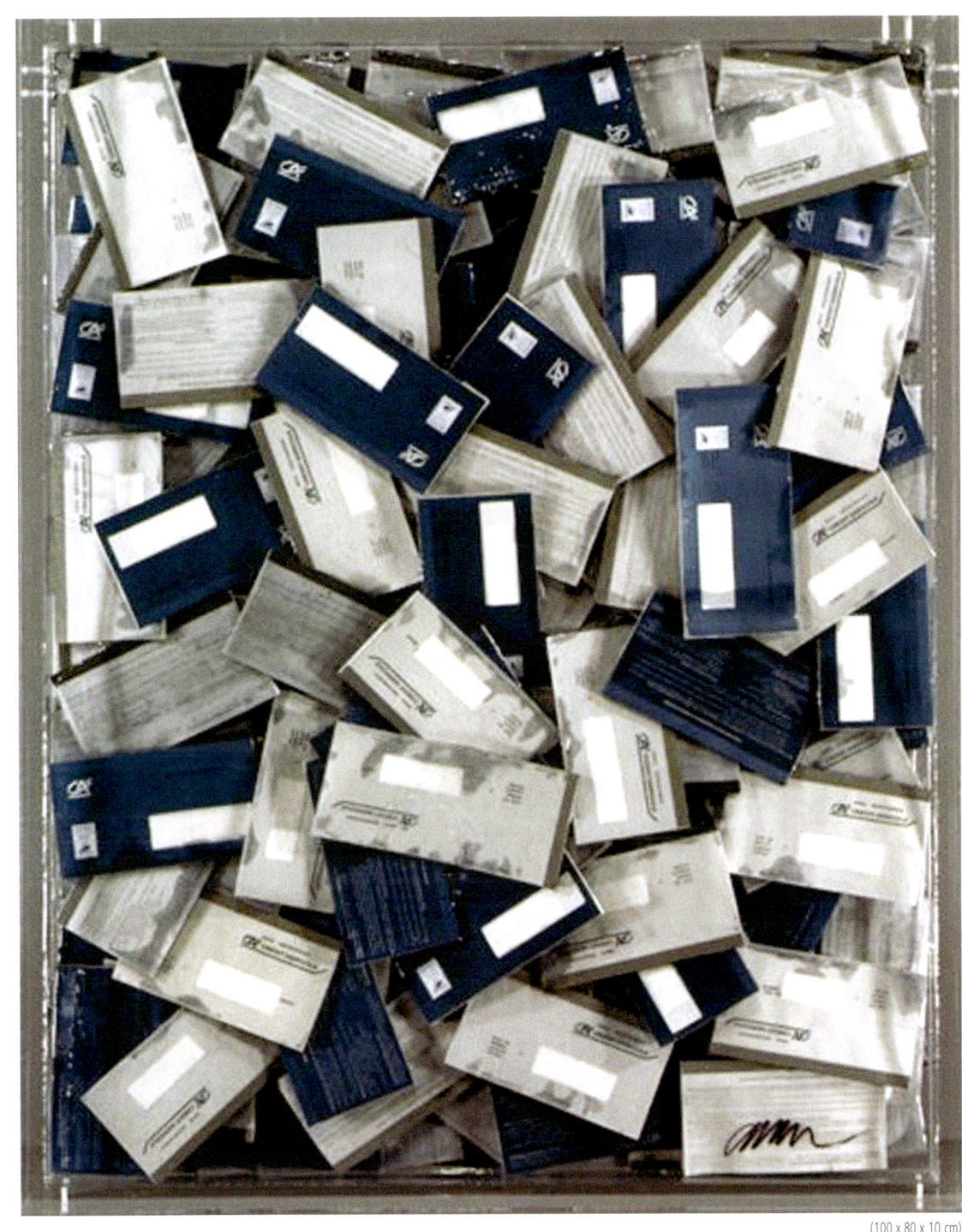

Arman
Untitled (1998)

(100 x 80 x 10 cm)

Depression and Society

Sébastien Mehal
Level for a Man Author of Light (2004)
(290 x 250 cm)

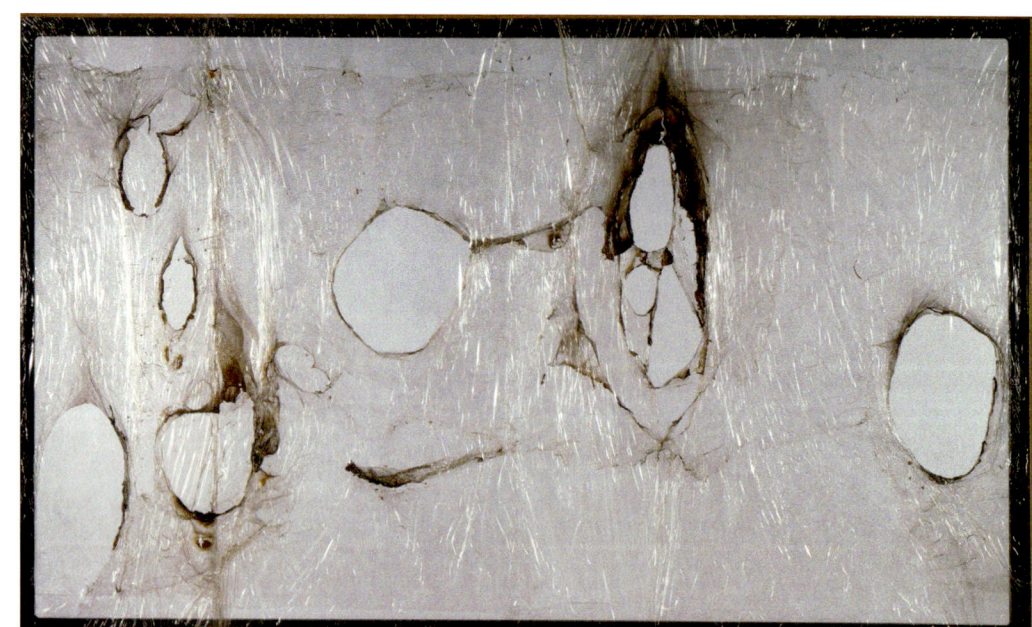

Alberto Burri
Combustione plastica (1964)
(2.510 x 1.505 m)

Focussing now on the qualities that could be assigned to depression, what immediately comes to mind is to speak of solitude, disenchantment, slowness, paralipsis and helplessness and the feeling that it is too late, now. It is no mystery that our contemporary world is in the midst of a crisis regarding its values insofar as the most established dogmas are being questioned either because they have demonstrated their limits or because they are disqualified by the very principle that nothing lasts. So it is that every day we are faced with absurd scenes of destruction and plunged at the same time into a powerful feeling of helplessness. This negative information feeds – in us, as in the depressed person – a form of nostalgia for the past, remembered as more glorious than it actually was. Above all, however, it is the quick obsolescence of objects, the furtiveness of human relations and the emergency of survival behaviour that generates in our societies a sensation of solitude in the middle of an anonymous multitude.

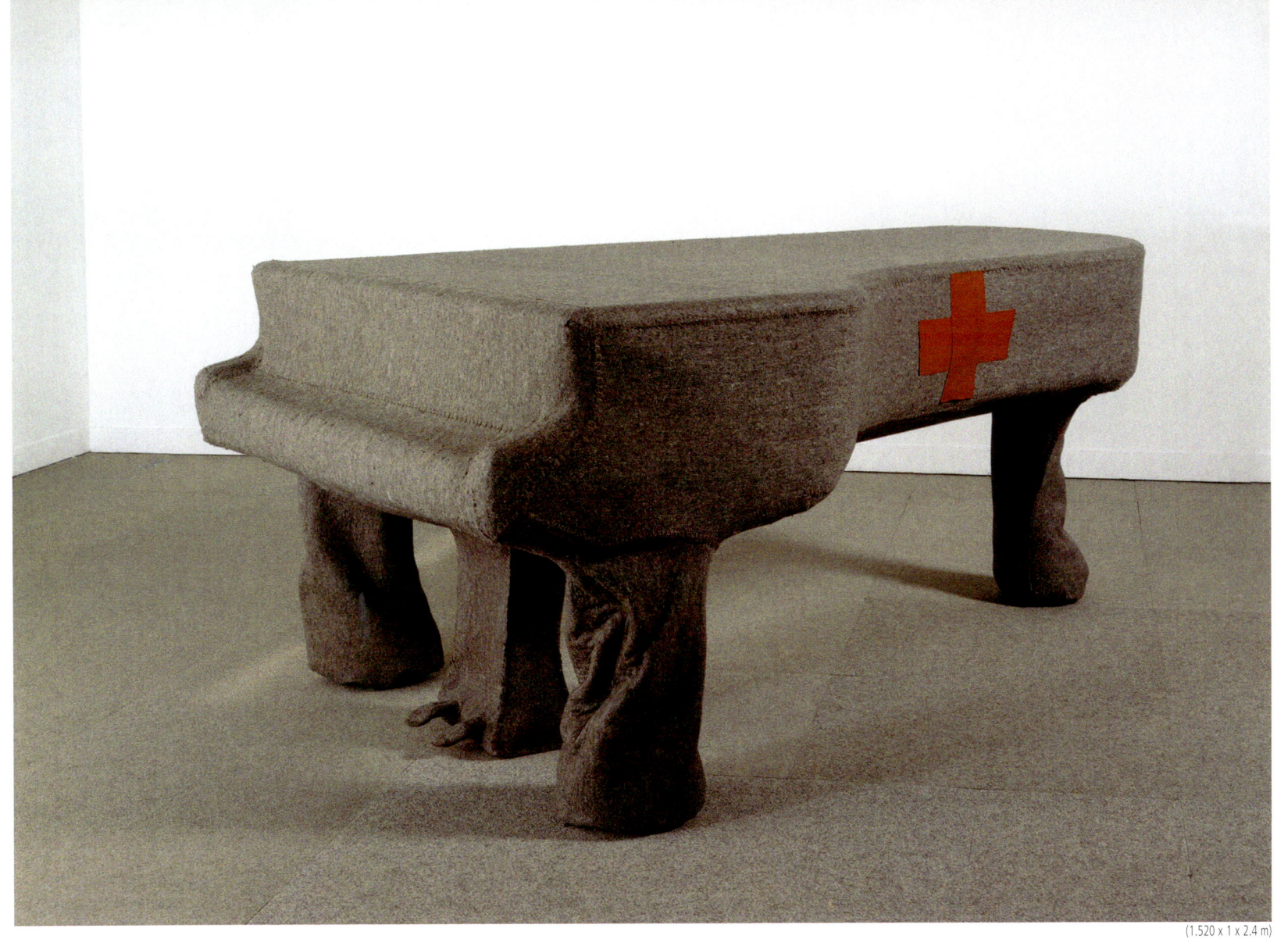

(1.520 x 1 x 2.4 m)

Joseph Beuys
Homogenous Infiltration for Grand Piano (1994)

By showing in their work the disenchantment, the helplessness and the inanity of our daily life, certain artists will solicit in us an emotion that is echoed by a pessimistic analysis of our modernity. The work of Alberto Burri, constituted of charred plastic materials, or of Joseph Beuys with his piano packed in felt, hence inaudible as well as unplayable, is suggestive of the rapid expiration of everyday objects. These latter, having also fallen ill, display the red cross of the help they can no longer provide. The plastic artist Sébastien Mehal in his silent, minimalist and enigmatic work also signifies solitude and raises the question of meaning.

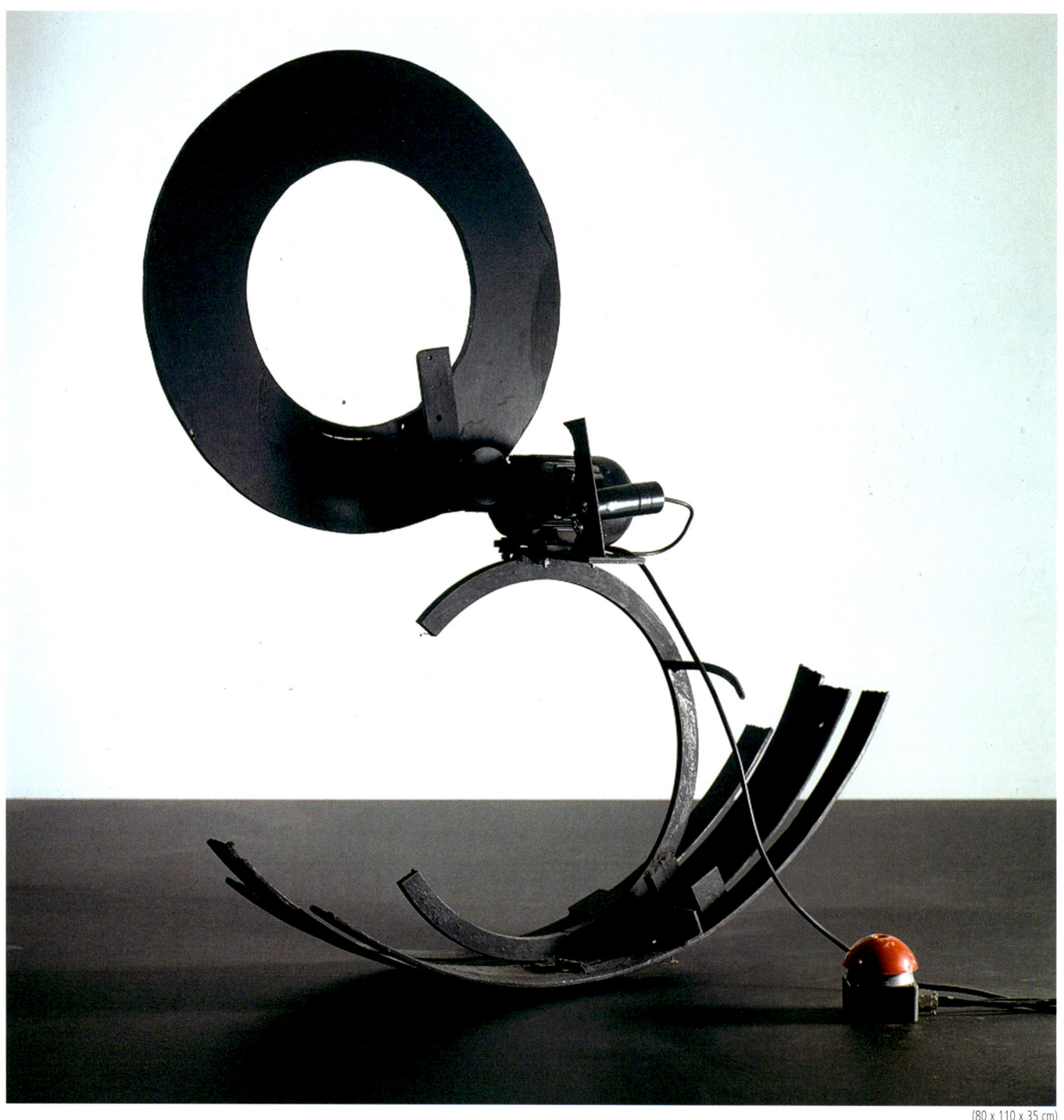

(80 x 110 x 35 cm)

Jean Tinguely
Santana (Bascule) (1966)

Recurrence and Society

The third pillar of bipolar disorder, recurrence, can be assimilated in turn with cyclicity, repetition and more of the same despite apparent change. There is no doubt that the abundance of information and forms in our everyday life includes a large part of repetition of the same forms and the same data in just barely different clothing. Whether we are in the area of advertisement, dress codes or ideas, we are often in the presence of infinite variations of identical representations. Oscillating between obsession – in its reassurance function – and recurrence – for lack of creative power – repetition has progressively invaded our contemporary world, in which innovations are either not heard or co-opted and repeated until they are desubstantiated. As in bipolar disorder, the repetition we are describing seems to be as absurd as it is unavoidable. Suggesting the vision of a world filled increasingly and daily with ineluctable repetitions, the work of certain contemporary artists questions us on our capacity to free ourselves from hypnosis and become creators ourselves. Thus, the unceasing oscillation of Jean Tinguely's bascules – just as Bruce Nauman's work, particularly that for which he uses *looped videos* – is emblematic of repetition pushed to the extreme. Drained of their explicit meaning, messages are saturating our understanding without, however, providing any matter for us to craft our own answers.

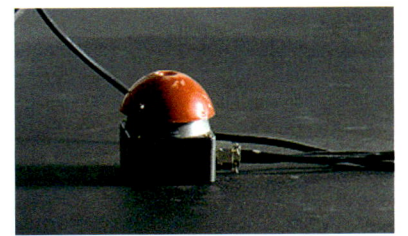

References

1. Akiskal, H.S., "Classification, Diagnosis and Boundaries of Bipolar Disorders: A review", in *Bipolar Disorder*, edited by Maj, M., Akiskal, H.S., Lopez-Ibor, J.J. and Sartorius, N., John Wiley, Chichester, England, 2004.
2. Angst, J.,"The Course of Affective Disorders", *Psychopathology* 19 (Suppl 2): 47-52, 1986.
3. Aretaeus of Cappadocia, *On the Causes and Indications of Acute and Chronic Diseases*, translated by F. Adams, London, The Sydenham Society, 1856.
4. Baillarger, J., "De la folie à double forme", *Annales Médico-psychologiques*, 1854, t. VI, 368.
5. Bourdieu, P., *Le sens pratique*, Paris, Éditions de Minuit, 1980.
6. *DSM-IV - American Psychiatric Association: Diagnostic and Statistical Manual of Mental Disorders*, 4th edition, Washington, D.C., American Psychiatric Association, 1994.
7. Falret, J-P., *De la folie circulaire*, Bull, Académie de médecine, 1854, t. XIX, 382.
8. Goodwin, G., Sachs, G., *Bipolar Disorder*, Fast Facts, Health Press, Oxford, 2004.
9. Goodwin, G., *Mood Disorder in Companion to Psychiatric Study*, 7th Edition, Johnstone, E.C., Cunningham Owens, D.G., Lawrie, S.M., Freeman, C.P.L., Editors, Churchill Livingstone, Edimburgh, 2004.
10. Kraepelin, E., *Dementia Praecox and Manic-Depressive Insanity*, The Classics of Psychiatry and Behavioral Sciences Library, New York, 1989.
11. Kraeplin, E., *Psychiatrie*, Leipzig, Barth, 1909-1915, 8th edition, 4 volumes.
12. Leonhard, K., *The Classification of Endogenous Psychoses*, translated by Berman, R. John Wiley and Sons, Inc., New York, N.Y., 1979.
13. Lévi-Strauss, C., *Anthropologie structurale*, Paris, Plon, 1958.
14. Perris, C., "A study of bipolar (manic-depressive) and unipolar recurrent depressive psychoses", I. Genetic investigation, *Acta Psychiatr Scand.*, 1966, Suppl 194:15-44.
15. Postel, J., Quetel, C., *Nouvelle histoire de la psychiatrie*, Dunod, Paris, 1982.
16. Sedler, M., "Falret's Discovery: the Origin of the Concept of Bipolar Affective Illness", *American Journ Psychiatry* 140: 1127-1133, 1983.
17. Weygandt, W., 1899a., *Uber die Mischzustande des Manisch-Depressiven Irreseins*, J.F. Lehmann, Munich. Translation in Marneros, A., "Origin and development of concepts of bipolar mixed states", *J Affect Disord.*, 2001 Dec. 67 (1-3): 229-40, Review.
18. Winokur, G., "Unipolar Depression: Is It Divisible into Autonomous Subtypes?" *Arch Gen Psychiatry* 36: 47-52, 1979.

Index of Artists

Guillaume Apollinaire (1880-1918), 44, 45

Arman (Arman Fernandez) (born in 1928), 76, 77

Matthew Barney (born in 1967), 6, 7

Joseph Beuys (1921-1986), 78, 79

Pierre Bonnard (1867-1947), 49, 50, 51

Fernando Botero (born in 1932), 12, 13

Alberto Burri (1915-1995), 78, 79

Sophie Calle (born in 1953), 46, 47

Sandro Chia (born in 1946), 64, 65

Robert Combas (born in 1957), 58, 59

Erró (Gudmundur Gudmundsson) (born in 1932), 30, 31

Katharina Fritsch (born in 1956), 40, 41

El Greco (Domenikos Theokopoulos) (1541-1614), 70, 71

Matthias Grünewald (1475-1528), 28, 29

Andreas Gursky (born in 1955), 68, 69

Thomas Hirschhorn (born in 1957), 52, 53

David Hockney (born in 1937), 10, 11

Alain Jacquet (born in 1939), 38, 39

Frida Khalo (1910-1954), 60, 61

René Magritte (1898-1967), 56, 57

Henri Matisse (1869-1954), 48, 50, 51

Sébastien Mehal (born in 1970), 78, 79

Claude Monet (1840-1926), 14, 15

Bruce Nauman (born in 1941), 72, 73

Orlan (born in 1947), 36, 37

Pierre Roy (1880-1950), 16, 17

Niki de Saint-Phalle (1930-2002), 34, 35

Jean-Jacques Sempé (born in 1932), 62, 63

Kiki Smith (born in 1954), 24, 25

Jean Tinguely (1925-1991), 80, 81

Vincent van Gogh (1853-1890), 8, 9

Jean-Pierre Velly (1943-1990), 20, 21

Bill Viola (born in 1951), 22, 23

Linde Wächter-Lechner (born in 1944), 26, 27

Psychiatry Index

Agitation, 30, 68, 73

Antipsychiatry, 75

Anxiety, 9, 10, 16, 24, 28, 35, 38, 41, 71

Body, 12, 23, 24, 28, 35, 36, 56

CIM-10, 66

Cognition, 10, 14, 16, 20, 23, 24, 28, 30, 36, 38, 41, 44, 46, 51, 63, 68, 71, 73

Cotard's syndrome, 35, 36

Curative treatment, 26

Cut off from ordinary perception, 6, 9, 10, 12, 20, 23, 24, 28, 35, 38, 68, 71

Death ideas, 20, 35, 60, 71

Delusion, 23, 35

Depressive state, 9, 20, 24, 28, 35, 41, 60, 71

Drug or alcohol abuse, 43

DSM-IV, 66

Dual Form Insanity, 18, 19

Emotional changes, 6, 23, 30, 38, 41, 73

Euphoria, 12, 30, 73

Exuberant, extravagant behaviour, 12, 30, 36, 44, 56, 59

Genetics, 67

Grandiosity, 9, 10, 12, 23, 30, 59, 63, 68

Guilt, worthlessness, 24, 28, 35, 41, 60

Hallucination, 9, 23

History, 32, 33

Hopelessness, 16, 20, 24, 28, 35, 41, 60, 71

Hypomania, 41

Language, 36, 44, 73

Manic and depressive states, 6, 14, 16, 23, 26, 30, 36, 46, 51, 53, 64

Manic state, 10, 12, 38, 44, 56, 59, 63, 68, 73

Melancholy, 20, 28, 35, 60, 71

Mental pain, 20, 24, 28, 35, 71

Mixed states, 12, 30, 54, 59

Omnipotence, 10, 14, 23, 30, 44, 63, 68

Physical complaints, 24, 35, 36

Preventive treatment, 6, 16, 26, 64

Psychosis, 9, 23

Psychotherapy, 46, 58

Rapid cycling, 43

Relapse, 6, 16, 26, 64

Sadness, 20, 24, 28, 35, 41, 61, 71

Self esteem (loss of), 20, 24, 28, 35, 60

Sexual drive (increased), 56

Social consequences, 9, 10, 12, 44, 51, 53, 64, 68

Sociological approach, 74

Solitude, 12, 14, 16, 20, 23, 24, 28, 35, 51, 60, 71

Structuralism, 75

Suicide, 60, 71

Support from people, 53

Talkativeness, 44, 73

Thought (racing), 10, 36, 42, 73

Unity of the Self, 38, 10, 46, 68, 73

Vulnerability, 16, 26, 53

Withdrawal from others, 10, 12, 14, 23, 24, 28, 35, 51, 60, 68, 71

Photo Credits

Pages 6-7: Barney, Matthew: Cremaster 4 (1994). Production still © 1994 Matthew Barney Photo: Michael James O'Brien, Courtesy Gladstone Gallery.

Pages 8-9: van Gogh, Vincent : Starry Night / *Nuit étoilée* (1889). New York, Museum of Modern Art (MoMA) © 2005, Digital image, The Museum of Modern Art, New York/Scala, Florence. Oil on canvas, 73.7 x 74.3 cm. Acquired through the Lillie P. Bliss Bequest.

Pages 10-11: Hockney, David: The steering wheel (1982). Photocollage, 75 x 91 cm. © All rights reserved.

Pages 12-13: Botero, Fernando: Ballerina / *Danseuse à la barre* (2001). Oil on canvas, 309,9 x 386,7 cm. © Fernando Botero.

Pages 14-15: Monet, Claude : Woman with Umbrella Turned to the Left / *Essai de figure en plein air : femme à l'ombrelle tournée vers la gauche* (1886). Musée d'Orsay, Paris. © Photo RMN / © Hervé Lewandowski. Oil on canvas, 88 x 131 cm.

Pages 16-17: Roy, Pierre: Danger on the Stairs (1927 or 1928). New York, Museum of Modern Art (MoMA). © Adagp, Paris 2005 – © 2005, Digital image, The Museum of Modern Art, New York/Scala, Florence. Oil on canvas, 91.44 x 60 cm. Gift of Abby Aldrich Rockefeller.

Pages 20-21: Velly, Jean-Pierre: Period. Nothing more (1978). © Héritiers J.P. Velly - Photo www.velly.org Francesco Allegretto. Burin, aqua fortis, dry-point on chine appliqué, ed. Don Quichotte, Rome 1978 (100 copies). Copper, 345 mm x 490 mm.

Pages 22-23: Viola, Bill: Going Forth By Day (2002), "First light". Video/sound installation. Photo: Kira Perov.

Pages 24-25: Smith, Kiki: Dream/*Sueño* (1992). New York, Museum of Modern Art (MoMA) © 2005, Digital image, The Museum of Modern Art, New York/Scala, Florence. © Kiki Smith and Universal Limited Art Editions, courtesy Pace Editions, Inc.,New York. Etching and aquatint on handmade Japanese paper, composition: 59.53 x 125.09 cm; sheet: 106.20 x 195.8 cm. Publisher and printer: Universal Limited Art Editions, West Islip, NY. Editions: 33. Gift of Emily Fisher Landau.

Pages 26-27: Wächter-Lechner, Linde: Earth Song / *Le chant de la terre* (1990). © Courtesy of Linde Wächter-Lechner. 19,5 x 100 x diametre: 31 cm.

Pages 28-29: Grünewald Matthias: The Crucifixion, Issenheim Altarpiece / *La Crucifixion, Retable d'Issenheim* (between 1512 and 1516). © Musée d'Unterlinden – F 68000 COLMAR Photo O. Zimmermann. 458.5 x 336 cm.

Pages 30-31: Erró (known as), Gudmundur Gudmundsson: Miss America (1997). © Collection Laurent Strouk © Photo: Courtesy of Erró. 195 x 130 cm.

Pages 34-35: Saint-Phalle, Niki (de): Gilles de Rais (1964). © Adagp, Paris 2005 - © 2005 NIKI CHARITABLE ART FOUNDATION, All rights reserved, Photo Credit: Laurent Condominas. Objects, painting, wire, 125 x 80 x 37 cm.

Pages 36-37: Orlan: Disfiguring-Refiguring : Pre-Columbian Hybridization No. 14 / *Refiguration/Self-hybridation précolombienne n° 14* (1998). © Adagp, Paris 2005 – Courtesy of Galerie Michel Rein, Paris. Aluminium-backed Cibachrome, 99.89 x 149.86 cm. (100 x 150 cm).

Pages 38-38: Jacquet, Alain: Portrait of a Woman, Jeannine / *Portrait de femme, Jeannine* (1965). © Adagp, Paris 2005. Acrylic on canvas in two parts, 130 x 195 cm each.

Pages 40-41: Fritsch, Katharina: Company at the Table / *Tischgesellschaft* (1988). © Adagp, Paris 2005 – Photo: Courtesy of Matthew Marks Gallery, New York. Polyesther, wood, cotton, paint 141 x 1600.04 x 172.72/198.12 cm.

Pages 44-45: Apollinaire, Guillaume : The Tie and the Watch / *La cravate et la montre,* Calligrammes, 1966, nrf (1st ed 1925). © Éditions Gallimard.

Pages 46-47: Calle, Sophie: The Tie / *La cravate* (1996). Reconstitution of a room with objects from «Autobiographical Stories». © Adagp, Paris 2005 – photo: Courtesy of Galerie Emmanuel Perrotin, Paris / Miami.

Pages 48, 50: Matisse, Henri: French Window in Collioure / *Porte-fenêtre à Collioure* (September-October 1914). © Succession H. Matisse – © Photo CNAC/MNAM Dist. RMN / © Philippe Migeat. 1.165 m x 89 cm.

Pages 49-50: Bonnard, Pierre: Studio with Mimosa / *L'atelier au mimosa* (1939 - October 1946). © Adagp, Paris 2005 – © Photo CNAC/MNAM Dist. RMN / © Philippe Migeat. 1.275 x 1.275 m.

Pages 52-53: Hirschhorn, Thomas: United Nations Miniature (2000). Miniature representation on the ground of 10 regions in conflict in the world (Rwanda, Sierrra Leone, Congo, Kosovo, Bosnia, Chechnya, East Timor, Lebanon, Palestine/Israel, Chiapas). Cardboard, wood, tape, plastic, aluminum paper, spray paint, desk lamp, painted toys, artificial plants, books, photocopies, printed matter. Variable dimensions (approx. 120 m^2). Created for the Lyons Biennial. © Adagp, Paris 2005 – Photo Courtesy of Galerie Chantal Crousel © Florian Kleinefenn. Collection Museo de Arte Contemporaneo de Castilla y Leon – MUSAC.

Pages 56-57: Magritte, René: The Rape / *Le viol* (1945). © Adagp, Paris 2005 – © Photo CNAC/MNAM Dist. RMN / © Christian Bahier / Philippe Migeat. 65.3 x 50.4 cm.

Pages 58-59: Combas, Robert: Denise's robe / *Le peignoir à Denise* (1994). © Adagp, Paris 2005 – photo : Art Unlimited Amsterdam.

Pages 60-61: Kahlo, Frida: The suicide of Dorothy Hale (1939). (59,7 x 49,5 cm). © 2005 Banco de México Diego Rivera & Frida Kahlo Museums Trust. Av. Cinco de Mayo No. 2, Col. Centro, Del. Cuauhtémoc 06059 México, D.F. © Phoenix Art Museum, Arizona – Photo The Library Art Museum.

Pages 62-63: Sempé: drawing from *Sauve qui peut*, 1972, © Éditions Denoël et Sempé, 1964.

Cover, pages 64-65: Chia, Sandro: The Idleness of Sisyphus (1981). New York, Museum of Modern Art (MoMA). © Adagp, Paris 2005 – © 2005, Photo Scala, Florence. Oil on canvas, in two parts, 309.88 x 386.71 cm. Acquired through the Carter Burden, Barbara Jakobson, and Saidie A. May Funds and purchase.

Pages 68-69: Gursky, Andreas: Madonna 1 (2001). © Courtesy of Monica Sprüth Galerie, Köln / Adagp, Paris 2005 – © Photo CNAC/MNAM Dist. RMN / © Georges Meguerditchian. 275 x 200 cm.

Pages 70-71: El Greco: View of Toledo (1597). The Metropolitan Museum of Art. H.O. Havemeyer Collection, Bequest of Mrs H.O. Havemeyer, 1929. (29.100.6) Photograph © 1992 The Metropolitan Museum of Art. 121.3 x 108.6 cm.

Pages 72-73: Nauman, Bruce: Eat/Death (1972). Neon, 19.1 x 64.1 x 5.4 cm). © Adagp, Paris 2005 – Photo © Stedelijk Museum Amsterdam.

Page 77: Arman (Arman Fernandez, known as): Untitled / *Sans Titre* (1998). Accumulation of cheque books (Crédit agricole) in a box made of plexiglass, 100 x 80 x 10 cm. © Adagp, Paris 2005 – Photo: Courtesy of Arman Studio.

Page 78: Mehal, Sébastien: Level for a Man Author of Light / *Hauteur d'homme auteur de lumière* (2004). Acrylic on canvas, 290 x 250 (diptych). © Sébastien Mehal (www.mehal.net).

Page 79: Beuys Joseph: Homogenous Infiltration for Grand Piano / *Infiltration homogen für Konzertflügel* (1994). Felt- and cloth-covered piano, 1.52 x 1 x 2.4 m. Musée national d'Art moderne – Centre Georges Pompidou, Paris. © Adagp, Paris 2005 – © Photo CNAC/MNAM Dist. RMN / © Adam Rzepka.

Page 79: Burri, Alberto: *Combustione plastica*, 1964. Charred polyvynil (2.510 x 1.505 m). Musée national d'Art moderne – Centre Georges Pompidou, Paris. © Fondazione Palazzo Albizzini "Collezione Burri", Città di Castello © Photo CNAC/MNAM Dist. RMN / © All rights reserved.

Pages 80-81: Tinguely, Jean: Santana (Bascule) (1966). 80 x 110 x 35 cm. Donation Niki de Saint-Phalle. Museum Tinguely, Basel. © Adagp, Paris 2005 – © Photo Christian Baur, Bâle.

Acknowledgments

John Libbey Eurotext would like to extend its special appreciation for their help in the completion of this work to:
Pierre Higonnet (www.velly.org) and Arthur Velly
Erró and Laurent Strouk
Orlan

Philippe Nuss thanks each of his patients. Their sensitivity, the finesse of their descriptions and the quality of their therapeutic involvement have afforded him a better approach and understanding of the mental world of bipolar disorder. He also wishes to testify gratitude and debt to his friend and master, Prof Maurice Ferreri, for the rigor and the wealth of his clinical observations as well as for the freedom and creativeness of his thought.

The authors thank Marina Urquidi for her precise and sensitive translation into English. Her availability and her involvement supported them throughout the writing of this book.

Date of printing October 2005, Corlet Imprimeur, S.A. - N° 86949